Meal Prepping for Weight Loss

By

Emma Krieger

Contents

Introduction

As they say, once you start meal-prepping, you never go back....or something like that. If you've never been much of meal-prepper, my hope is that this book converts you. I honestly don't know how I'd manage if I didn't plan and prepare all my meals in advance each week.

Let's face it. We're all busy. Weeknights are tough. Most of us don't have the desire or energy to spend our last waking hours in the kitchen every night preparing food when we could easily pick up some take-out on the way back from work. Or maybe we'll just stock up on those tv dinners and stash them in our freezers—even thouh we know most of this dishes aren't very nourishing and they're loaded with chemicals and preservatives. It gets old quick, doesn't it?

Maybe you resolved to yourself to cook more, then on a given weeknight, you find yourself staring blankly into your fridge wondering what to make without sufficient energy or inspiration to make a decision. As the pizza boxes pile up, and the owners of the local Mexican restaurant start to know you by name because you're their new best customer, you might find that your waistline starts to grow. You might also find that your bank account starts to dwindle. Maybe that's why you bought this book. You want better for yourself.

Or maybe you're a busy mom and just want to be able to make the most of your time and prepare healthy meals for your family. Whatever your situation, this book will arm you with inspiration. I tried to pack this book with recipes for every occasion. Light simple meals, fancier comfort foods, grab and go breakfasts, side dishes, homemade salad dressing and EVEN desserts. That's right, I have an entire section on healthy desserts that you can make ahead.

So what exactly is meal prepping: it's similar to meal planning in the sense that you should have a menu set in mind and do your grocery shopping so you have all the necessary ingredients on hand, but with the added advantage that you make food in bigger batches so it can serve as multiple meals so you don't have to cook every day. The other advantage is that you can make a dish ahead for a later day. For example: if you know on Thursday you have a meeting after work and simply won't have time to prepare anything, you can make something on Wednesday when you have extra time, and then problem solved. Thursday is already taken care of. There's also a **Freezer Meals Section** in this book which you might find very helpful. I love to always stock up on at least 5 or 6 homemade freezer meals so I always have a fallback option.

So what to expect from this book?

- I've only included delicious recipes. I didn't bother with anything that was healthy but bland—because what's the point? No one wants to eat that.
- All of the recipes contained in this book are low in calories, trans fats, sugars and other harmful nutrients. All the recipes are healthy and nutritious carefully designed to help you pursue a healthy lifestyle
- All of the recipes contain:
  - Detailed instructions for how to prepare the dish
  - Detailed instructions for what you need to do to prep the dish ahead, and then what you need to do just before eating
  - Information on how long you can store the dish for
  - Serving amounts
  - Photos of the food
  - Detailed nutrition information

How Does Meal Prepping aid in weight loss?

Apart from the obvious point that it keeps you from resorting to eating out in restaurants and falling back on fattening unhealthy take out options and "instant meals" or "frozen tv dinners," it also helps you with portion control

If you prep a dish, you'll portion it out so you already are containing the amount you're eating. Pairing it with a healthy low calorie side dish will help you feel fuller without eating more.

The recipes in this book borrow from some of the world's best diets including:

- The low carb/keto diet
- The Paleo Diet
- The Mediterranean Diet
- The Asian Diet
- The Vegan Diet
- The Vegetarian Diet
  .

All of these diets have proven effective in improving health and aiding in weight loss. This book will vanquish the myth that eating healthy means you have to eat boring or tasteless food. It sounds too good to be true, but it's not: not only will you thoroughly enjoy the dishes you prepare from this book, but you'll start seeing the pounds drop off as you experiment with these different eating/cooking styles.

You'll have no problem driving right past the Mexican restaurant or deleting the pizza delivery company's number out of your phone if there's already a delicious healthy meal prepared and waiting for you. You'll save money, you'll save a significant amount of time, and best of all, you'll feel good about what you're eating and you'll see serious results with your health and weight.

Cheers to living well and eating healthy! Now let's get on with the recipes.

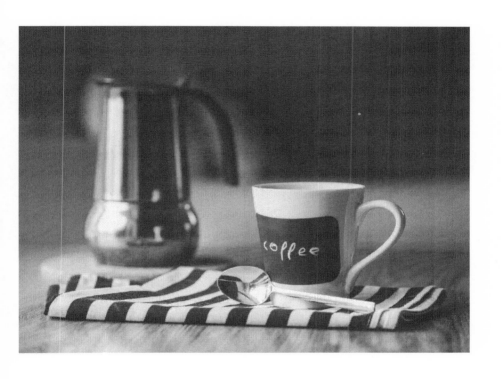

Grab & Go
Breakfast

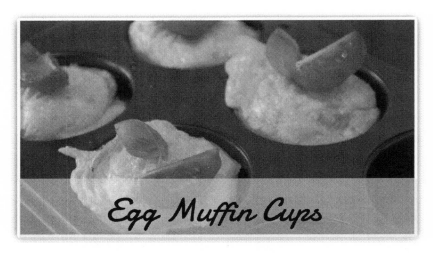

Egg Muffin Cups

SERVES 6 | PREP 5 MIN | COOK 20 MIN | READY IN 25 MIN

INGREDIENTS

A dozen cage-free eggs
1 red onion
1 green pepper
1 red pepper
1 jalapeño pepper (optional, for a spicy kick)
½ teaspoon pepper
½ teaspoon paprika
Olive oil (for cooking)

PREPPING

After baking the muffins, store them in the fridge for up to 4 days. When you're ready to eat, remove from the fridge and microwave or, slice the muffin in half and toast it in the toaster.
I like to serve it with salsa or guacamole.

NUTRITION PER SERVING:

Calories: 145, Fat: 8.9g, Carbs: 5.2g, Fiber: 1.2 g, Protein: 11.7 g.

DIRECTIONS

1. First, preheat your oven to 350 degrees. While your oven is preheating, begin chopping up the vegetables. Finely dice the red onion and peppers. If you do not want the spicy kick, you don't have to add the jalapeño pepper. Place all of the peppers in a bowl.
2. When all of the vegetables are cut, pour some olive oil into your cast iron skillet. Once the oil is hot, add the onions (first) and peppers (second) into the cast iron skillet and cook until done. Pro tip: if you want your food to be spicier, but don't have enough jalapeño peppers, add them in later. The rawer these jalapeño peppers are, the spicier they will be. If you cook them too much, they will lose some of their kick.
3. Crack all of the eggs and put them into a large bowl. Begin slowly whisking these so the yokes mix well with the egg whites. Make sure to not add oxygen into the mixture by beating the eggs. This process must be done gently. After your onions and peppers are sautéed, let them cool for a few minutes. Add these guys to your eggs.
4. Coat a muffin pan with olive oil. Fill these muffin cups with your eggs and cooked vegetables.
5. Cook them in the oven for 10 to 15 minutes. Remember, eggs do not need to be cooked too much or they will become gray and hard. All you need to do is make sure that the bacteria is burned away from the eggs. A great way to tell when this has happened is to see if the eggs are becoming fluffy and golden brown in the oven. This means that the muffins are fully cooked and you can remove them from the oven.

Note: the serving size is 2 muffins. This recipe will make 12 muffins, so if you are only cooking for 1, you may want to reduce the amounts to make less per batch since they only keep for 4 days.

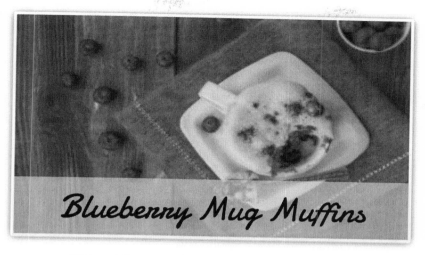

Blueberry Mug Muffins

Serves 4 | Prep 5 min | Cook 5 min | Ready in 10 min

INGREDIENTS

½ c. applesauce
4 tbsp Greek Yogurt
4 eggs
1 teaspoon vanilla extract
4 Tbsp, Honey
½ c. flour, (I use almond, but you can use any type you prefer)
1 tsp. baking powder
¼ tsp of salt
2/3 c. fresh Blueberries

DIRECTIONS

1. Whisk Together wet ingredients in a bowl (oil, applesauce, yogurt, eggs, vanilla and honey)
2. In a separate bowl, mix together the flour baking powder and salt. Then slowly combine the wet and dry ingredients and stir until combined so there are no lumps.
3. Stir in the blueberries but do not overmix or stir too vigorously to keep the blueberries intact

PREPPING

Store the blueberry muffin batter in an airtight glass or metal container in the fridge.
Each morning for the next 4 mornings, pour ¼ of the batter into a large, microwave-safe mug that you have sprayed with cooking spray
Microwave for about 1 minute. You may want to start with 50 seconds and check.
Alternatively: you can portion the batter out into 4 mugs right after you make the batter, and cover with plastic wrap or foil. Then the morning of, just remove the plastic or foil and microwave and enjoy.

Nutrition Per Serving:

Calories: 345, Fat: 18.5g, Carbs: 37.7g, Fiber: 1.4 g, Protein: 8.7 g.

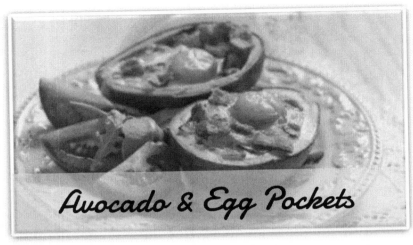

Avocado & Egg Pockets

SERVES 4 | PREP 10 min | COOK 20 min | READY in 25 min

INGREDIENTS

2 ripe avocados, pitted and halved
4 large eggs
kosher salt
Freshly ground black pepper
4 slices bacon

DIRECTIONS

1. Fry the bacon until quite crispy.
2. Slice the avocados in half, remove the pit

Prepping

Crack an egg into the center of the avocado halves where the pit was, and bake uncovered on a cookie sheet at 350 for 20 minutes
Remove from the oven and wrap each avocado pocket in foil. Refrigerate for up to 3 days, and store the bacon in foil at room temperature.
The morning of, microwave the avocado pocket until hot and crumble 1 of the slices of bacon on top.
Eat with a spoon scooping out part of the avocado and part of the egg together.

Nutrition Per Serving:

Calories: 267, Fat: 22.3g, Carbs: 8g, Fiber:6 g, Protein: 11.5 g.

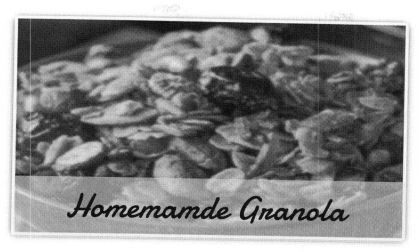

Homemamde Granola

SERVES 12 | PREP 15 min | COOK 35 min | READY in 65 min

INGREDIENTS

4 cups oats
1/2 c. unsalted almonds, chopped
1/2 c. walnuts, chopped
2 teaspoons ground cinnamon
½ tsp. dried ginger powder
1 teaspoon sea salt
1/4 c. flax seed
1/4 c. honey
1/4 c. vegetable oil
2 tsp vanilla extract
1/2 cup chopped dried cranberries
1/2 cup unsweetened shredded coconut

DIRECTIONS

Mix together oats, salt, cinnamon, ginger, and flax seed
In another bowl, mix together honey, oil, and vanilla. Then add the wet mixture to the dry. Spread the mixture into a deep glass baking dish that has been greased with cooking spray

Prepping

Bake uncovered for 25 minutes at 350, stirring occasionally. Then add the coconut, stir and bake for 5-10 more minutes. Once the granola has cooled slightly, stir in the dried cranberries. Once the granola is room temperature, pour it into a large freezer bag and store in the freezer. This will keep for quite a while in the freezer and keeps the nuts and fruit very fresh.
Before eating, measure out a serving of the granola and serve with almond milk and fresh fruit if desired.

Nutrition Per Serving:

Calories: 271, Fat: 15.4g, Carbs: 28.5g, Fiber:5.3 g, Protein: 6.5 g.

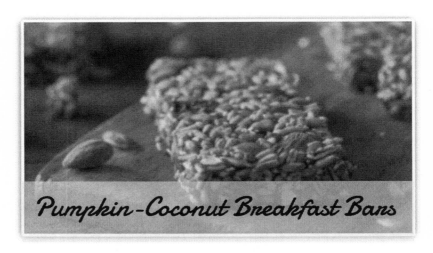

Pumpkin-Coconut Breakfast Bars

Serves **8** | Prep **15** min | Cook **20** min | Ready in **35** min

INGREDIENTS

1 cup oats
1 teaspoon baking soda
1 teaspoon baking powder
½ teaspoon salt
1 cup vanilla protein powder
1/3 c. coconut flakes, unsweetened
1 tbsp pumpkin pie spice
1/4 cup maple syrup or honey
1 cup pumpkin puree (from a can)
½ cup coconut milk
2 tbsp. water
½ c. pumpkin seeds

DIRECTIONS

In a bowl, mix together dry ingredients (oats, baking soda and powder, salt, protein powder, coconut flakes, and pumpkin pie spice). Mix until well combined
In a separate bowl, combine the pumpkin puree, honey and coconut milk and water
Mix together wet and dry ingredients and spread into a square baking dish that has been lined with waxed or parchment paper and then sprayed with cooking spray.
Bake at 350 for about 18-20 minutes

Prepping

When the pan has cooled, slice the bars into 8 even squares. You can store at room temperature in an air tight plastic container. Or for longer-term storage, place the bars in a plastic ziplock in the freezer. Just grab one out and allow it to thaw slightly before consuming as needed.

Nutrition Per Serving:

Calories: 197, Fat: 10.2g, Carbs: 20.7, Fiber: 3 g, Protein: 8.1 g.

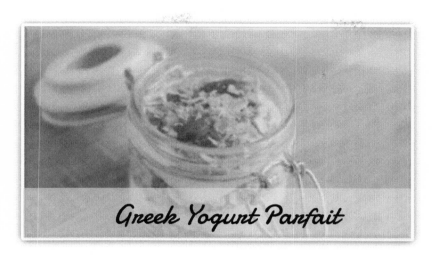

Greek Yogurt Parfait

Serves | Prep 5 min | Cook 0 min | Ready in 5 min

INGREDIENTS

2 C. unsweetened greek yogurt
3/4 c. Wholegrain granola (unsweetened)
¼ c. dried dates, chopped
1/8 c. almonds toasted, slivered
4 tsp. honey

DIRECTIONS

Put 1/4c. yogurt in the bottom of the jar or glass, then add a small amount of granola, another 1/4c. yogurt, a bit more granola, then top with dates, almonds and drizzle with 1tsp. honey
To keep the everything fresh, we recommend only assembling right before eating.

Prepping

Just have the ingredients on hand and pre-measured. Then the morning of, you simply have to toss the ingredients together in a jar. The Reason I don't recommend assembling the parfaits ahead of time, is because the granola can get soggy, and nobody wants that..

Nutrition Per Serving:

Calories: 178, Fat: 8.7g, Carbs: 31.5, Fiber: 3.4 g, Protein: 15.9 g.

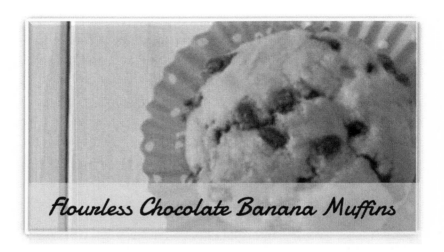

Flourless Chocolate Banana Muffins

Serves 12 | Prep 10 min | Cook 20 min | Ready in 30 min

INGREDIENTS

3 large or 4 medium bananas, ripe
4 eggs
2/3 c. natural peanut butter
1/4 c. honey
3/4 tsp. baking powder
1/2 tsp. vanilla extract
¼ c. dark chocolate chips (at least 70% cacao)

DIRECTIONS

Throw everything except the chocolate chips into the blender. Pulse until smooth and mixed
Line 12 muffin tins with papers and lightly spray them with cooking spray
Evenly pour the batter into the tins and then sprinkle the chocolate chips on top and stir them into the batter slightly with a spoon.
Bake at 400 for 15-18 minutes or until toothpick comes out clean

PREPPING

Once the muffins have cooled, place them in a freezer bag and put them in the freezer. Take the muffins out as needed and heat in the microwave, or slice in half and heat in the toaster

Nutrition Per Serving:

Calories: 170, Fat: 9.5g, Carbs: 17.8, Fiber: 1.8 g, Protein: 6.2 g.

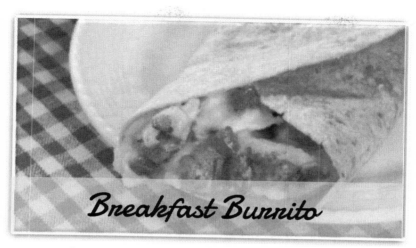

Breakfast Burrito

Serves 10 | Prep 15 min | Cook 10 min | Ready in 25 min

INGREDIENTS

1 lb. reduced fat breakfast sausage
1 bell pepper, diced
1 onion, diced
12 eggs
1/4 cup milk
Kosher salt and fresh cracked pepper.
2 Tbs vegetable oil
2/3 c. shredded mozzarella
10 100% whole-grain tortillas
Spinach (optional)
Hot Sauce (optional)

PREPPING

To assemble, evenly portion out the cooked sausage, scrambled eggs, peppers and onions, and cheese across the 10 whole wheat tortillas. Roll up the tortillas tucking in the sides so that they are snuggly and securely rolled. Place the burritos in a large freezer bag. Freeze & microwave as needed and enjoy.

DIRECTIONS

In a medium skillet, brown the breakfast sausage draining off the fat until fully cooked and crumbly. (If the sausage is pre-seasoned, you don't need to do anything, otherwise, season to taste)

Remove the sausage from the skillet. And toss in the peppers and onions. Sauté for several minutes until the onions become translucent and the peppers are soft.

In a large bowl, crack in 12 eggs. I recommend first cracking them into a small bowl and then adding them to the large bowl. This reduces the risk of ruining the whole mixture with a bad egg or getting shells in the eggs. Whisk the eggs with the milk

Using the sausage pan, scramble the eggs until they've reached desired doneness. If the pan doesn't have enough grease from the sausage, you can lightly spray cooking spray on it to keep the eggs from sticking

Nutrition Per Serving:

Calories: 236, Fat: 14.1 g, Carbs: 13.4g, Fiber: 1.9 g, Protein: 14.2 g.

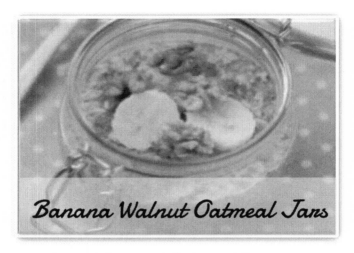

Banana Walnut Oatmeal Jars

Serves 1 | Prep 5 min | Cook 5 min | Ready in 10 min

INGREDIENTS

1/2 cup rolled oats
1/4 cup dried bananas
2 tbsp. roughly chopped walnuts
1 Tbsp. flax seeds (or chia)
1/2 tsp. Cinnamon
Fresh banana slices (optional)
1 Tbsp Honey

DIRECTIONS

In a mason jar, combine oats, dried bananas, walnuts, flax, and cinnamon. Shake until combined

Prepping

Fill as many mason jars as desired with the dry ingredients. And store on a shelf until ready for use.
The morning of, pour in 2/3 cup boiling water. Stir and set until desired consistency. Top with fresh bananas and honey.

Nutrition Per Serving:

Calories: 385, Fat: 14.2 g, Carbs: 58.4, Fiber: 8.6 g, Protein: 9.4 g.

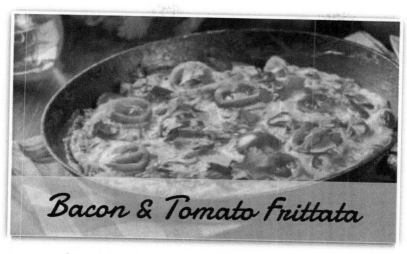

Bacon & Tomato Frittata

Serves 6 | Prep 10 min | Cook 20 min | Ready in 30 min

INGREDIENTS

A dozen fresh eggs
Olive oil (for cooking)
1/3 pound of grass fed bacon
(more or less 6 slices)
5 to 6 Roma tomatoes
1 red onion
2 cloves of garlic
3 tablespoons of your
favorite leaves (basil, parsley,
etc.) or mix and match
Half a teaspoon of sea salt
(optional)

PREPPING

Slice the frittata into 6 pie slices, wrap in foil
and store in the fridge
When ready to eat, heat in the microwave
(without the foil) or in the oven, keeping it
wrapped in foil

Nutrition Per Serving:

Calories: 201, Fat: 13.1g, Carbs:
6.8, Fiber: 1.6 g, Protein: 14.9 g.

DIRECTIONS

1. Preheat your oven to 350 degrees Fahrenheit. While your oven is preheating, crack the dozen eggs and begin to whisk them together. Remember to never season your eggs right away—they will turn gray by the time you serve them if you do. Mince your garlic, cut your tomatoes into circles, and cut up the red onions. Keep these separate from the eggs and bacon for now. Later on, we will combine them..

2. Cut your bacon into tiny strips and cook in your cast iron skillet. Cook on the stove with olive oil until the bacon looks crispy. Once cooked, place the bacon on a separate plate. Use the same olive oil to then cook the minced garlic and onions.

3. Once the minced garlic and onions are cooked, add the bacon to the mix. Then add the eggs. Eggs do not need to be cooked very quickly, so the pan doesn't need to be super hot. Once you see that the eggs are beginning to take shape, place the circular tomato slices on top of the frittata. Cool down the meal for a few minutes, making sure that the tomatoes do not sink to the bottom of the egg concoction.

4. Next begin cooking this frittata in your already pre-heated oven for 20 minutes. Set a timer for 10 minutes. Once the timer goes off, sprinkle in the leaves over the frittata. Because they are least dense, these leaves will be the first to cook, and you don't want to burn them, so always make sure to add them at the end.

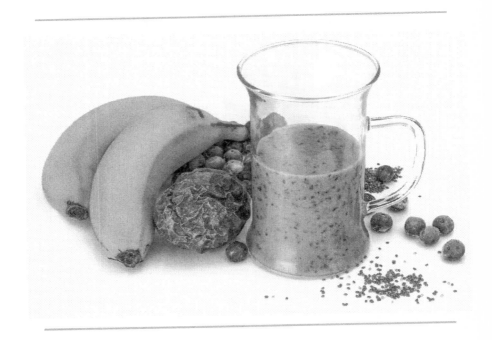

Smoothies

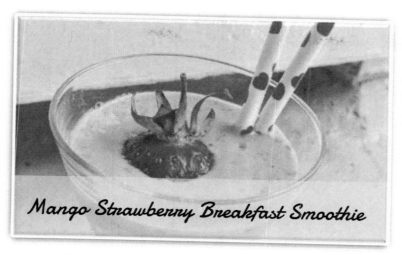

Mango Strawberry Breakfast Smoothie

Serves 4 | Prep 10 min | Cook 0 min | Ready in 10 min

INGREDIENTS

DIRECTIONS

1 banana
1 cup frozen strawberries
1 cup frozen mango
1 cup Greek yogurt
1/2 cup almond milk (or soy or cow)
1/4 tsp. ground cinnamon (optional)

Combine all ingredients in blender and pulse until smooth and completely blended.

Prepping

you can make this smoothie ahead and store in a glass jar in the fridge for up to 3 days, or freeze it for even longer, and eat it like ice cream for a frozen treat. You'll want to allow it to thaw slightly before consuming.

Nutrition Per Serving:
Calories: 171, Fat: 8.4g, Carbs: 20, Fiber: 2.9 g, Protein: 6.4 g.

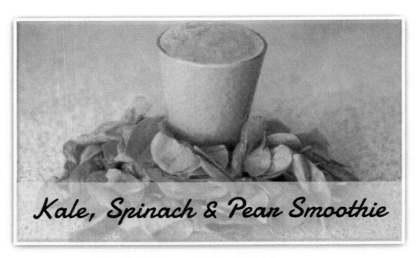

Kale, Spinach & Pear Smoothie

Serves 4 | Prep 10 min | Cook 0 min | Ready in 10 min

INGREDIENTS

2 cups spinach
2 cups kale leaves
1 pear
2 bananas
3 cups almond milk
3 tablespoons honey

DIRECTIONS

Chop up the spinach and kale leaves. Combine them in a blender and add almond milk. Once the leaves are fully blended with the almond milk, chop up the pear and bananas.
Add them to the blender. Once blended, drizzle honey for sweetness and continue to blend until smooth. Enjoy and refrigerate the leftovers for the next day.

Prepping

you can make this smoothie ahead and store in a glass jar in the fridge for up to 3 days

Nutrition Per Serving:
Calories: 223, Fat: 3g, Carbs: 45.4, Fiber: 4.4 g, Protein: 7.3 g.

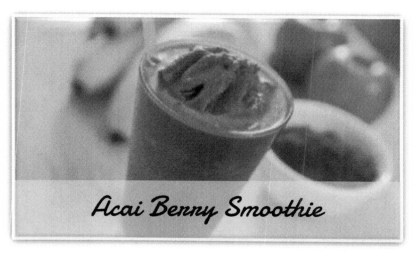

Acai Berry Smoothie

Serves 4 | Prep 10 min | Cook 0 min | Ready in 10 min

INGREDIENTS

2 medium bananas
2 cup acai berries
1 cup strawberries
½ cup blueberries
¼ cup coconut milk

DIRECTIONS

Chop up the bananas and put them in a food processor. Cut leaves off the strawberries and add to the bananas. Add blueberries and acai berries. Finally, add the coconut milk.

Prepping

Blend the ingredients together for 1 minute or until smooth. Refrigerate leftovers for two to three days.

If you're packing to take to work, you can either just make it and portion it into cups and mugs or just bring the ingredients at the beginning of the week and if your office has a blender, you can just blend before drinking.

Nutrition Per Serving:

Calories: 163, Fat: 4.3g, Carbs: 33.3, Fiber: 5.3 g, Protein: 2.1 g.

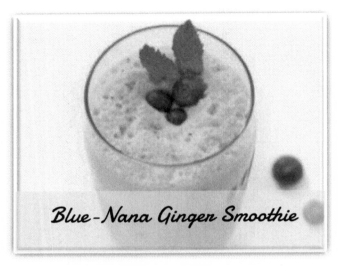

Blue-Nana Ginger Smoothie

Serves 4 | Prep 10 min | Cook 0 min | Ready in 10 min

INGREDIENTS

2 bananas, sliced
1 c. blueberries
1 c yogurt
3 Tbsp honey
1 tsp freshly grated ginger

DIRECTIONS

Throw everything into a blender and pulse until smooth

Prepping

you can make this smoothie ahead and store in a glass jar in the fridge for up to 3 days, or freeze it for even longer, and eat it like ice cream for a frozen treat. You'll want to allow it to thaw slightly before consuming.

Nutrition Per Serving:
Calories: 166, Fat: 1.1g, Carbs: 36.3, Fiber: 2.5 g, Protein: 4.5 g.

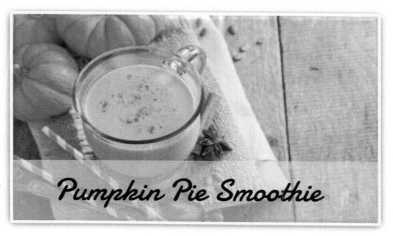

Pumpkin Pie Smoothie

Serves 4 | Prep 10 min | Cook 0 min | Ready in 10 min

INGREDIENTS

1 1/2 cup almond milk
3 tsbp. honey
1 1/2 cup pumpkin puree
2 apples, cored and choppd
3 tsp. pumpkin pie spice

DIRECTIONS

Throw everything into a blender and pulse until smooth. Top with a sprinkle of cinnamon.

PREPPING

you can make this smoothie ahead and store in a glass jar in the fridge for up to 3 days, or freeze it for even longer, and eat it like ice cream for a frozen treat. You'll want to allow it to thaw slightly before consuming.

Nutrition Per Serving:
Calories: 191, Fat: 2.2g, Carbs: 45.2, Fiber: 6.1 g, Protein: 4.4 g.

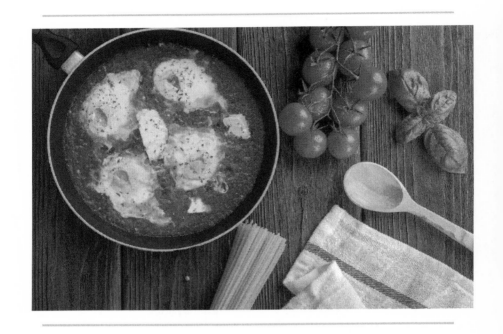

Mediterranean Diet Dishes

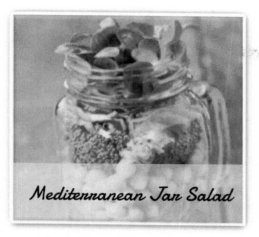

Mediterranean Jar Salad

Serves 4 | Prep 10 min | Cook 0 min | Ready in 10 min

INGREDIENTS

1 cup dry quinoa
½ teaspoon salt
Fresh ground pepper
1/3 cup olive oil
1 tablespoon red wine vinegar
2 garlic cloves, minced
½ teaspoon dry crushed basil
½ teaspoon dried crushed thyme
3 cups fresh greens of your choice (baby spinach, arugula etc)
1 15 oz can chickpeas
¼ c. black olives, sliced,
1 cucumber, diced
Cherry Tomatoes (optional)
1 cup raw broccoli florets
Fresh Basil (optional)

DIRECTIONS

Cook quinoa following package directions
In a small bowl, mix together salt, pepper, oil, vinegar, basil, and thyme.

Prepping

In the bottom of 4 mason jars, evenly portion out the chickpeas, olives, and cucumbers. Then portion out the dressing you mixed together in the previous step pouring over the chickpeas
Add a layer of cooked quinoa (after it's cooled), then last, top with the greens.
Seal Jar and store in the fridge for up to 4 days
Top with tomatoes before eating if desired

Nutrition Per Serving:
Calories: 359, Fat: 20.8 g, Carbs: 37.5, Fiber: 8.3 g, Protein: 10.4 g.

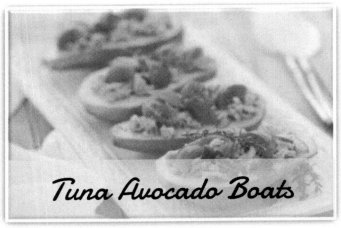

Tuna Avocado Boats

Serves 4 | Prep 15 min | Cook 0 min | Ready in 15 min

INGREDIENTS

2 (6oz) cans of Tuna
4 tbsp. Olive oil Mayo
¼ c. red onion, chopped
2 Stalks of Celery, chopped small
1 tsp. Balsamic vinegar
Salt and Pepper
2 medium avocados

DIRECTIONS

Drain the tuna and combine in a small bowl with all other ingredients except avocado. When ready to serve, halve the avocado, remove the pit and stuff ¼ of the tuna mixture into the center. Garnish with more red onion and tomato slices if desired

Prepping

Portion the tuna salad into 4 small containers. The morning of, slice the avocado and squeeze lemon juice on it to keep it from turning brown.
Bring the avocado half and the tuna to work with you and assemble before eating. The tuna mixture can keep up to 3-4 days in glass in the fridge.

Nutrition Per Serving:
Calories: 233 Fat: 13.4 g, Carbs: 4.7, Fiber: 3.2 g, Protein: 22g.

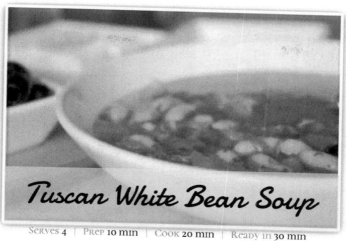

Tuscan White Bean Soup

Serves 4 | Prep 10 min | Cook 20 min | Ready in 30 min

INGREDIENTS

2 cups shredded chicken (yield from a whole chicken cooked and bones/skin removed)
1 large carrot, sliced into rounds
1 large leek, sliced into rounds
2 tsp. Extra Virgin Olive Oil
½ tsp. sage
½ tsp. Italian Seasoning
Salt and Pepper
28 oz. Chicken Broth
1 (15 oz) can of Cannellini Beans
2 c. Water

DIRECTIONS

Heat oil in a large pot and salute leeks and carrots until they become tender (about 4 minutes).

Add seasonings and salt and pepper and stir and cook for 1 minute longer.

Add all remaining ingredients and stir until well combined.

Cook until flavor is to your desired taste.

PREPPING

Store in glass in the fridge for up to 3 days. Heat on the stove top or in the microwave before eating.

Nutrition Per Serving:
Calories: 231 Fat: 5.5 g, Carbs: 19.6, Fiber: 6.6 g, Protein: 25.1 g.

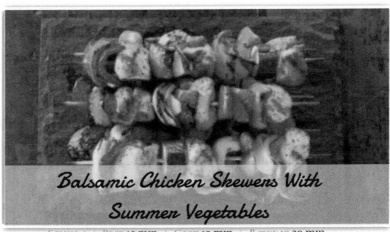

Balsamic Chicken Skewers With Summer Vegetables

Serves 4 | Prep 10 min | Cook 10 min | Ready in 30 min

INGREDIENTS

1/4 cup balsamic vinaigrette
1/4 cup barbecue sauce
1 teaspoon Dijon mustard
1-1/2 lbs chicken breast, cut into 1 in. cubes & seasoned w/salt & pepper
2 cups cherry tomatoes
2 bell peppers chopped in large chunks
1 large zucchini chopped into rounds

DIRECTIONS

Soak the skewers in water for a few minutes

In a small bowl, whisk together, the BBQ sauce, Dijon Mustard, and Balsamic Vinaigrette. Set aside a small amount for dipping later.

Marinate the chicken cubes in this sauce and mix to coat the chicken cubes.

Load the skewers with the vegetables and chicken alternating

Grill for several minutes on each side until the chicken is fully cooked and vegetables get grill marks.

Serve with the extra sauce that did not touch the raw chicken.

Prepping

Make the skewers and store in the fridge on plates with foil for up to 2 days.
Grill before eating.

Nutrition Per Serving:

Calories: 255, Fat: 9.4 g, Carbs: 15.7, Fiber: 3.1 g, Protein: 26.4 g.

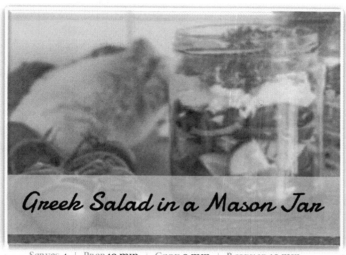

Greek Salad in a Mason Jar

Serves 4 | Prep 10 min | Cook 0 min | Ready in 10 min

INGREDIENTS

1 can (15 oz) chickpeas
1 large cucumber, chopped
½ c. black olives sliced
2 Roma tomatoes, diced
1/4 cup red onion, sliced
3 tablespoons olive oil
1 tablespoon lemon juice
1/4 teaspoon salt
1/8 teaspoon pepper
5 cups torn mixed salad greens
1/2 cup crumbled feta cheese

DIRECTIONS

Whisk together the lemon, oil, salt and pepper in a small bowl.
Drain and rinse the chickpeas.

Prepping

portion out into 4 medium sized mason jars. Pour the olive oil mixture over the beans.
Then add the olives, cucumber, tomato and onion.
Then add the greens and top with Feta.
Store the jars in the fridge for up to 4 days. Shake well and toss before eating

Nutrition Per Serving:
Calories: 255, Fat: 17.7 g, Carbs: 19.9, Fiber: 5.2 g, Protein: 7.5 g.

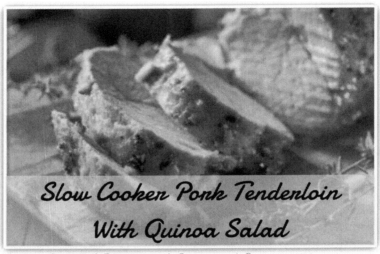

Slow Cooker Pork Tenderloin With Quinoa Salad

Serves 4 | Prep 30 min | Cook 3 HRS | Ready in 4 HRS

INGREDIENTS

¼ c. extra virgin olive oil
½ tsp. kosher salt
¼ tsp. freshly ground black pepper
1 lbs of pork tenderloin
1 cup chicken broth
4 garlic cloves, minced very fine
Salt and pepper
1 cup quinoa
2 tablespoons apple cider vinegar
1/2 cup minced fresh parsley
1/3 cup dried cranberries
1/4 cup sliced almonds, toasted

DIRECTIONS

1. Pour the chicken broth into the bottom of the slow cooker pan.
2. Season and pat the pork tenderloin with salt, pepper and half of the garlic then transfer into the slow cooker.
3. Cook about 2 hours on low or until meat thermometer reads 160 degrees. Then pull the pork out of the slow cooker and place it on a cutting board.
4. Pour the liquid in the slow cooker into a liquid measuring cup and pour back into the slow cooker 1 cup of the liquid. Add in the quinoa and cook on high for around 15 minutes or until the quinoa is cooked and fluffy. Add the cranberries and almonds and mix.
5. In a small bowl, whisk together oil, vinegar, ½ tsp. salt, and ¼ tsp. pepper, the rest of the garlic and the parsley. Whisk until the vinaigrette is well combined.
6. Slice the tenderloin and serve with the quinoa. Drizzle the vinaigrette over both.

PREPPING

Portion out into 4 medium sized mason jars. Pour the olive oil mixture over the beans.
Then add the olives, cucumber, tomato and onion.
Then add the greens and top with Feta.
Store the jars in the fridge for up to 4 days. Shake well and toss before eating

Nutrition Per Serving:
Calories: 474, Fat: 22.3 g, Carbs: 31.2, Fiber: 4.4 g, Protein: 36.7 g.

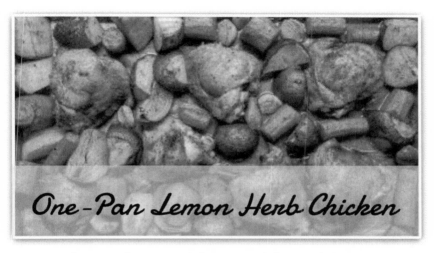

One-Pan Lemon Herb Chicken

Serves 4 | Prep 20 min | Cook 40 min | Ready in 60 min

INGREDIENTS

4 skin-on , bone-in chicken thighs
3 tablespoons olive oil
1 tablespoon red wine vinegar
1 lemon, juiced (about ¼ c fresh juice)
4 cloves garlic
1 tbps dired Italian Seasoning
1 tsp dried basil
Kosher Salt and Pepper
8 small red skinned potatoes, chopped into fourths
1 large onion, chopped
1 large zucchini , sliced
4 large Carrots, chopped into sticks

Nutrition Per Serving:

Calories: 459, Fat: 22.3 g, Carbs: 20.9, Fiber: 47.7 g, Protein: 24.8 g.

DIRECTIONS

1. In a small bowl, whisk together oil, vinegar, lemon juice, garlic, Italian seasoning, basil, salt and pepper. Pour half of this mixture into another container and set aside.
2. Pat chicken dry with paper towels, then place in the other half of the marinade in a large zip lock bag.
3. Marinate overnight if you can
4. Chop the vegetables and set them aside

Prepping

About 40 minutes before eating, preheat the oven to 400 degrees.
In a heavy bottomed skillet (cast iron if you have it) heat 1 tbsp. Remove the chicken thighs from the marinade and sear on both sides for 2-3 minutes or until golden brown.
Place the chicken on a large baking sheet surrounded by the chopped vegetables. Pour the other half of the marinade (not the one that's already touched the chicken) over the vegetables and stir them around until coated
Bake for 30-40 minutes or until vegetables are tender and slightly caramelized and chicken reads 165 degrees with a meat thermometer.
You can store the cooked finished dish in a glass container for up to 3 days in the fridge.

33

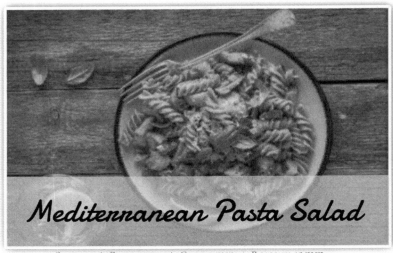

Mediterranean Pasta Salad

Serves 5 | Prep 15 min | Cook 0 min | Ready in 15 min

INGREDIENTS

1/2 red onion, diced
1 large cucumber, diced
1 cup grape tomatoes, sliced in half
½ cup kalamata olives, chopped
1/2 cup green olives, chopped
½ c crumbled feta cheese
2 oz hard salami, sliced into 1/2-inch thick rounds and then quartered
1/4 cup olive oil
2 cloves garlic, minced
1/8 cup balsamic vinegar
1 tsp honey
1 teaspoon kosher salt
1/2 teaspoon ground black pepper
½ lb of dried whole wheat or spinach pasta of your choice
Spinach (optional)

DIRECTIONS

1. Prepare the pasta according to the package instructions
2. After the past is cooked and drained and cooled, slightly, stir in the chopped tomatoes, cucumbers, black and green olives, feta, and salami.
3. In a small bowl, whisk together the oil, vinegar, honey, garlic, salt and pepper.
4. Pour the vinaigrette over the pasta mixture

Prepping

Store the pasta salad in a glass container in the fridge. This dish is best served cold (great as a lunch to pack and take to work, or as a light meal after a long day. I like to stir in a few handfuls of fresh spinach right before eating. If you do use spinach, don't add it until just before eating because it will get soggy and slimy.

Nutrition Per Serving:
Calories: **313**, Fat: 20.6 g, Carbs: 24.6, Fiber: 4.1 g, Protein: 11.1 g.

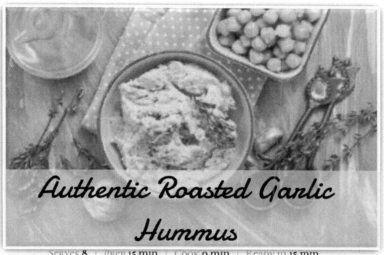

Authentic Roasted Garlic Hummus

Serves 8 | Prep 15 min | Cook 0 min | Ready in 15 min

INGREDIENTS

10 cloves garlic
2 tbsp. olive oil
2 1/2 cup canned chickpeas, rinsed and drained
¼ c. tahini
¼ c. fresh lemon juice
Salt
1 tsp za'atar, dried (you can get it at most large supermarkets, or any middle eastern or Greek stores)
Cayenne Pepper (optional)

DIRECTIONS

1. Chop or thinly slice the garlic cloves.
2. In a large skillet, heat 2 tbsp olive oil. Add the garlic cloves and allow them to brown slightly. Stir constantly and keep the heat on medium so that the garlic doesn't burn. Once the garlic is all golden or even slightly brown and tender, remove from heat.
3. Combine all ingredients in a food processor (except za'atar) and pour in the roasted garlic including the oil. Pulse and blend until the mixture is desired consistency. Add more lemon juice if you need more liquid, and add salt and pepper to taste as needed.

Prepping

Store in a glass container in the fridge for up to a week.
Serve with chopped veggies for a healthy snack or light lunch (carrots, broccoli, cucumber etc)
Top with Za'atar if you like the flavor, and mix in cayenne if you like it with a kick.

Nutrition Per Serving:
Calories: 167, Fat: 1.3 g, Carbs: 16.9, Fiber: 5.1 g, Protein: 6.2 g.

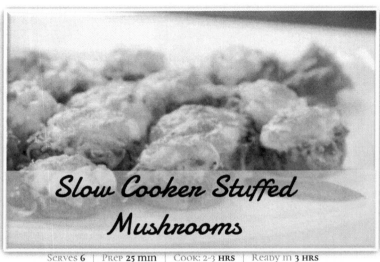

Slow Cooker Stuffed Mushrooms

Serves 6 | PREP 25 min | COOK: 2-3 HRS | Ready in 3 HRS

INGREDIENTS

2 (6oz.) packages mushrooms (white or Portobello) washed, stems removed, and caps set aside
1 tbsp. extra-virgin olive oil
2 cloves garlic, minced
1 (8 oz.) Neufchâtel (cream) cheese, at room temperature
1/4 cup freshly-grated Parmesan cheese
¼ - ½ tsp. kosher salt (to taste)
1/4 teaspoon ground black pepper
1/4 teaspoon onion powder
1/4 teaspoon ground cayenne pepper
1 c. chicken stock

DIRECTIONS

1. Chop mushroom stems until finely minced.
2. Heat oil in medium skillet on stove over medium heat. Add minced garlic and mushroom stems and sauté stirring constantly until mushroom stems are soft (about 2-3 minutes).
3. Once the garlic mixture has cooled slightly, combine it in a medium mixing bowl with the Neufchâtel cheese, parmesan cheese, salt, pepper, onion powder and cayenne pepper. Mix thoroughly until the mixture is completely combined
4. Use a spoon, carefully fill all the mushroom caps evenly with the cream cheese mixture
5. Layer the mushrooms in the bottom of the slow cooker. Add the chicken broth.

PREPPING

Cook for 2-3 hours on high. If desired, add more grated parmesan on top. You can also crisp up the tops of the stuffed mushrooms by placing them in the oven under the broiler for a minute or two.Great as an appetizer, or with some veggies or a green salad for a light vegetarian meal.

Nutrition Per Serving:
Calories: **206**, Fat: 17.7 g, Carbs: 6, Fiber: 1.3 g, Protein: 8.1 g.

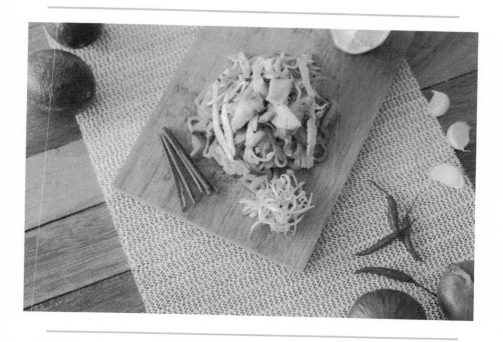

Healthy Asian Dinners

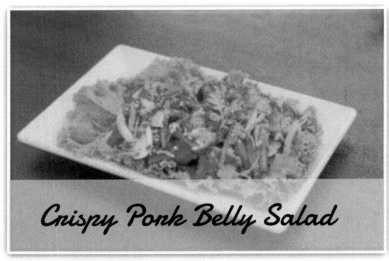

Crispy Pork Belly Salad

Serves 4 | PREP 30 min | COOK: 0 HRS | READY in 30 Min

INGREDIENTS

½ lb. of pork belly slices
2 pears, sliced
1 avocado
6 cups of salad leaves of your choice (rocket goes well with pear...)
2 tsp of salt
1/2 cup of chopped almonds
2 tbsp. honey
4 tsp of water
2 tsp of Dijon mustard
2 tsp of any whole grain mustard for the dressing
1/4 c. of rice wine vinegar
1/4 c. tsp oil

DIRECTIONS

1. Cover the pork with half of the olive oil. Cook in a hot oven until crunchy and browned, about 20 to 30 minutes.
2. Warm a pan and add the water and stevia to the pan, and add the walnuts once the stevia has dissolved. Cook for five minutes until the liquid has caramelised the walnuts.
3. Tip the nuts onto a tray and leave to cool. Note: they will be hot.
4. Chop the pear and cheese into bite-sized pieces.
5. Make the vinaigrette by adding the mustards, vinegar and oil into a bowl and mixing well.
6. By this time the pork should be cooked. Remove set aside to cool, then chop into bite sized chunks.
7. Toss the salad in the vinaigrette and add the pork, nuts, cheese and pear.

PREPPING

Prepare all ingredients in advance, and store in glass containers. If packing your lunch, the morning of, assemble your salad, in a container and put the dressing in a separate container. Measure out the ingredients in advance. Do any chopping; a squeeze of lemon juice will help the pear chunks to stay crisp.

Nutrition Per Serving:
Calories: 455, Fat: 39.2, Carbs: 20.5, Fiber: 4.7 g, Protein: 6.7 g.

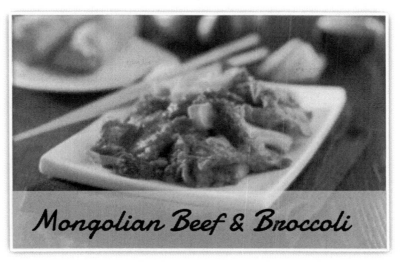

Mongolian Beef & Broccoli

Serves **6** | Prep **10 min** | Cook: **6 hrs** | Ready in **6 Hrs**

INGREDIENTS

2 lbs. chuck roast (or sirloin, or flank) chopped into 1-inch cubes
1/2 c. soy sauce
1 tsp. sesame oil
2 tbsp. hoisin sauce (optional)
1/4 tsp. fresh ground black pepper
1 c. beef stock
1 tbsp. brown sugar
1/2 inch fresh ginger, grated (about 2 tsps.)
3 cloves garlic, minced
1 (14 oz) bag frozen broccoli
1 large onion, rough chopped
Red pepper flakes (to taste)
1 tsp sesame seeds

DIRECTIONS

1.Combine all ingredients (except the sesame seeds) in the slow cooker. Cook on low for 5-6 hours or on high for 2-3 (or until beef is tender).

2. Sprinkle with sesame seeds and serve hot.

Prepping

Simply set the slow cooker to finish at your desired eating time, and then store leftovers in glass for up to 3 days. The leftovers make great packable lunches for the next few days.

Nutrition Per Serving:
Calories: **355**, Fat: **12.3**, Carbs: **12.9**, Fiber: **2.7 g**, Protein: **47 g**.

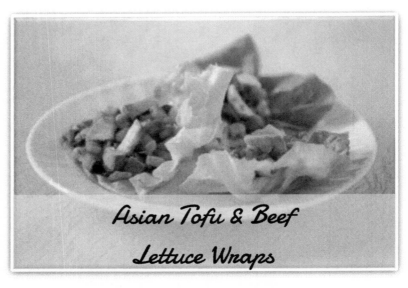

Asian Tofu & Beef Lettuce Wraps

SERVES 4 | PREP 20 MIN | COOK: 0 HRS | READY IN 20 MIN

INGREDIENTS

1 tbsp chili paste
1 tsp sesame oil
1/4 cup hoisin sauce
¼ cup soy sauce
2 tbsp. rice wine vinegar
8 oz tofu, cubed (about ½-1 inch)
3 inches fresh minced ginger (about 2 tbsp)
1 tbps canola oil
1/2 pound lean ground beef (90 percent or leaner)
1 avocado
1 large head Bibb lettuce, outer leaves discarded, leaves separated
1/4 cup chopped peanuts

DIRECTIONS

1. Whisk together chili, sesame, hoisin, soy sauce and vinegar in a small bowl.

2. Brown the beef in a large skillet and add the ginger and tofu stirring. Sauté until the ginger is fragrant and the tofu has been seared.

3. Stir in the sauce that you whisked together into the skillet. Simmer over medium low heat for about 3 minutes.

4. Remove from heat and allow to cool

PREPPING

Store the meat mixture in a glass container in the fridge for up to 4 days. Serve by scooping a spoonful of the beef mixture into the center of a bibb lettuce leaf and top with chopped avocado and peanuts. If you're packing these to take to work, don't assemble until right before eating. Keep lettuce separate.

NUTRITION PER SERVING:
Calories: 398, Fat: 23.8, Carbs: 19.6, Fiber: 6.1 g, Protein: 27.7 g.

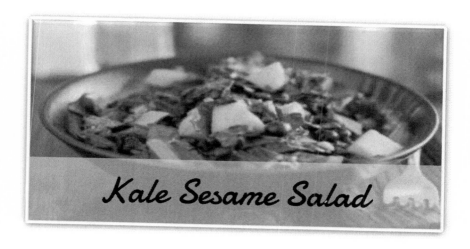

Kale Sesame Salad

Serves 4 | Prep 10 min | Cook: 0 hrs | Ready in 10 Min

INGREDIENTS

1 head of kale
1/2 tsp sea salt
1/8 c. lemon fresh lemon juice,
1 tbsp. olive oil
1 cup edamame beans, out of the pod
2-3 carrots chopped (about 1 cup)
1/4 cup sliced almonds, toasted
1 cup fresh mango, diced
¼ c. chopped scallions
1 tbsp sesame seeds

Dressing:
1 tsbp sesame oil
1 tbsp very finely minced ginger
1 tbsp olive oil
2 tbsp rice wine vinegar
2 tbps soy sauce
2 tsp honey

DIRECTIONS

1. In a small bowl, whisk together all of the dressing ingredients. Or to properly mix, pour all ingredients into a mason jar and tightly seal with a lid. Shake vigorously for at least 30 seconds to properly emulsify.

2. Roughly chop the kale after removing all the stems. Wash and pat dry with paper towels.

3. Add the rest of the salad ingredients on top of the kale

PREPPING

Store the salad (without the dressing) in a glass bowl covered with plastic for up to 2 days. Dress right before eating

Nutrition Per Serving:
Calories: 310, Fat: 18 g Carbs: 28.2, Fiber: 6.2 g, Protein: 12.7 g.

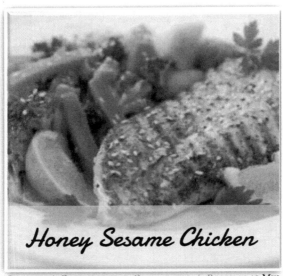

Honey Sesame Chicken

Serves 4 | Prep 10 min | Cook: 0 hrs | Ready in 10 Min

INGREDIENTS

3/4 cup chicken stock
1/3 cup honey
2 tablespoons sesame oil
1 1/2 tablespoons mustard
1 tbps Olive oil
4 chicken breast halves
Sea salt and ground pepper
3 teaspoons toasted sesame seeds
2 tablespoons sliced almonds
Lime Wedges

DIRECTIONS

1. Add the chicken stock with honey and sesame oil and mix until blended well. Then add mustard and stir. In your cast iron skillet, bring to a boil while whisking the mixture. Then lower the heat and cook until it has the consistency of honey. Set aside.

2. In you cast iron skillet, heat 1 tbsp. olive oil. Season chicken according to taste with salt and pepper. Add chicken to pan and cook for seven minutes searing on both sides. Check with meat thermometer to make sure it is fully cooked (at least 165 degrees F).

Prepping

Once your chicken is cooked, pour honey mixture over chicken, and sprinkle with sesame seeds. Any chicken that you would like to save, refrigerate. Do not pour honey onto chicken if you are not going to eat it that day. You can save the two parts of the meal if they are separate, but not together.

Nutrition Per Serving:
Calories: 366, Fat: 19.6 g Carbs: 26.1, Fiber: 1.3 g, Protein: 23.4 g.

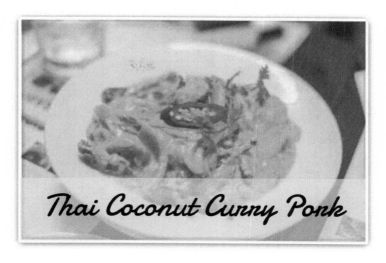

Thai Coconut Curry Pork

Serves 6 | Prep 10 min | Cook: 8 HRS | Ready in 8 HRS

INGREDIENTS

2 lb. pork shoulder, cut into 1-inch cubes.
1 red chili, seeds removed, minced (optional)
1/4 c. Thai yellow curry paste.
1 tbsp. fish sauce
1/2 tsp. ground cumin
1/2 tsp salt
2 medium onions, chopped
4 cloves of garlic, minced
2 tbsp. ginger, grated
1 cup of coconut milk
1-1/2 c. chicken stock
Fresh cilantro (optional)

DIRECTIONS

1. Combine all ingredients except cilantro in the slow cooker—mix until combined and pork cubes are evenly coated.
2. Cook on low for 8-10 hrs, or high for 4-5 hours.
3. Serve over brown rice

PREPPING

Simply set the timer of your slow cooker so that the dish is done when you're ready to eat. Store leftovers in glass in the fridge for up to 3 days. Reheat in the microwave.

Nutrition Per Serving:
Calories: 367, Fat: 28 g Carbs: 7.9, Fiber: 2 g, Protein: 21.7 g.

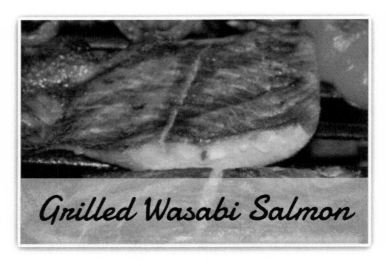

Grilled Wasabi Salmon

Serves 4 | Prep 10 min | Cook: 10 min | Ready in 20 min

INGREDIENTS

4 (6oz) salmon filets

2 cloves garlic, minced

2 tbsp soy sauce

1 teaspoon wasabi powder

2 tsp fresh ginger, minced

1/2 teaspoon dark sesame oil

½ tsp Salt

¼ tsp black Pepper

Fresh Lemon Wedges

DIRECTIONS

1. In a bowl, mix together the minced garlic and ginger, soy sauce, wasabi and sesame oil and salt and pepper.

2. Pour the marinade into a ziplock bag and add the salmon filets.

Prepping

You can marinate the fish overnight, then the next day when you're ready to eat, fire up the grill. Coat the grill with cooking spray if needed. Once the grill is hot, reduce the heat to medium and add the salmon filets searing and getting nice grill marks. Sear on both sides and cook for about 4 minutes on each side depending on the thickness of the fish or until the fish reaches the desired doneness.

Nutrition Per Serving:
Calories: 288, Fat: 12.7 g Carbs: 2, Fiber: 0.3 g, Protein: 38.5 g.

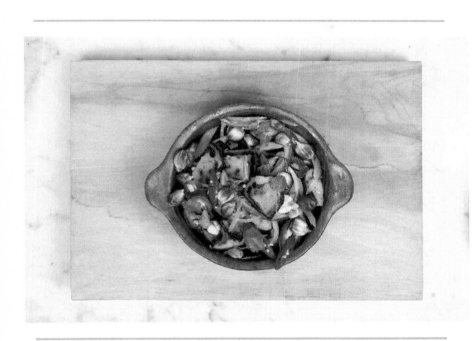

Healthy Dinners

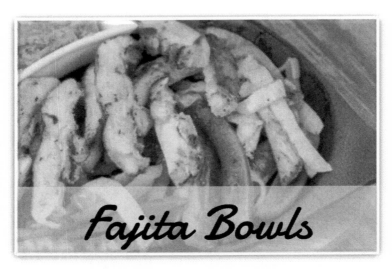

Fajita Bowls

Serves 4 | Prep 20 min | Cook: 10 min | Ready in 30 min

INGREDIENTS

1 pound boneless skinless chicken breasts cut into 1" cubes
1/4 teaspoon salt
½ teaspoon chipotle powder
½ tsp ground cumin
¼ teaspoon ground pepper
2 tbsp. Olive oil
1 medium red onion, sliced
1 green bell pepper, sliced
1 Yellow or Red bell peppe sliced
2 cups cooked brown rice
1 medium tomato, chopped
¼ cup chopped fresh cilantro
1 small jalapeno, chopped
1 (15 oz) can black beans, drained and rinsed

DIRECTIONS

1. Heat 1 tbsp of olive oil in a large skillet over medium heat. When the pan is hot, add the cubed chicken. Sprinkle on the salt, chipotle, cumin, pepper. Sitrring and pushing around the chicken so that its evenly coated with the spices
2. Cook for 5-7 minutes or until chicken is completely cooked. Remove chicken from the pan
3. Add another tbsp. of olive oil and toss in the onions, sliced peppers, and jalapeno. Season lightly with more salt and pepper. Stir fry until peppers are tender and onions are translucent.
4. While the vegetables are cooking, chop up the cilantro and mix it with the cooked rice in a separate bowl.

Prepping

In 4 microwave, safe containers, layer first the rice mixture, then chicken, then cooked peppers and onions, then ¼ of the black beans, then tomato. Cover the containers and store in the fridge for up to 4 days. Pop them into the microwave and heat and eat whenever you're ready. HINT: I love to squeeze fresh lime on right before eating—it really wakes up the flavors. Especially if the dish has been reheated.

Nutrition Per Serving:
Calories: 327, Fat: 10.9 g Carbs: 40.3, Fiber: 5.3 g, Protein: 18 g.

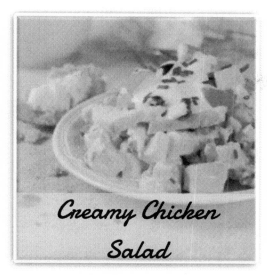

Creamy Chicken Salad

SERVES 6 | PREP 20 min | COOK: 20 min | READY in 45 min

INGREDIENTS

1 ½ lb boneless skinless chicken breast, cooked and diced into ½ inch cubes
1 cup dried cranberries
½ c. celery, diced
1 large green apple, cored and chopped
½ c. scallions chopped
1 cup plain, nonfat Greek yogurt
1/2 cup reduced fat mayonaisse
1 teaspoon kosher salt
1/2 teaspoon black pepper
1 tsp. dried tarragon
2 tbps. Fresh lemon juice
2 tablespoons fresh dill, chopped roughly
1/2 cup toasted almonds, slivered

DIRECTIONS

1. Cook the chicken (I like to poach the chicken: just place it in boiling water with carrots and onions and parsley. Remove and slice when the chicken is fully cooked and meat thermometer reads 165 degrees F.)
2. Once chicken is room temperature, combine all ingredients in a large bowl EXCEPT for the almonds

PREPPING

Portion the chicken salad out into 6 equal portions in Tupperware or glass. Keep almonds separate. Top with almonds right before eating.

Note: this can make a great light dinner or a very easy packed lunch. Enjoy the chicken salad in a whole wheat wrap, or on top of some salad greens, or in an avocado boat, or simply by itself.

NUTRITION PER SERVING:
Calories: 233, Fat: 7.3 g Carbs: 15.1, Fiber: 3.4 g, Protein: 27.4 g.

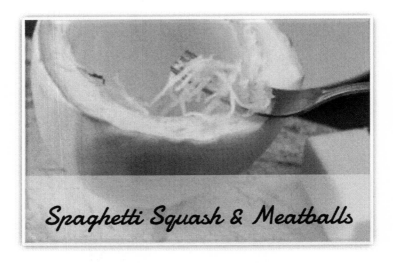

Spaghetti Squash & Meatballs

Serves 6 | Prep 30 min | Cook: 3-7HRS| Ready in 4 HRS

INGREDIENTS

1 tbsp. extra virgin olive oil
1 large Spaghetti Squash
1 (14.5 oz) jars of fire roasted diced tomatoes
2 c. Pomodoro sauce (plain marinara)
4 cloves garlic, minced
1 large yellow onion, diced
2 tsp. dried Italian seasoning
1 tsp. dried basil
1/2 tsp. dried oregano
Kosher salt and fresh black pepper to taste
1/4 tsp. fennel seeds (optional)
Red pepper flakes (optional)
20 frozen meatballs
1/4 c. fresh grated parmesan cheese

Nutrition Per Serving:
Calories: 305, Fat: 17.6 g Carbs: 24.1, Fiber: 3.4 g, Protein: 20.7 g.

DIRECTIONS

1. In a skillet over medium heat, heat the olive oil. Sauté the onions for 5 minutes, then add the garlic and cook for 2 more minutes stirring. Make sure nothing is sticking to the bottom of the pan. Add the fire roasted tomatoes, the pomodoro and all the herbs and spices. Stir until everything is incorporated and reduce heat to medium low, leave for 15 minutes with the lid propped.
2. Cut the spaghetti squash in half and remove the seeds and the stringy pulp (be careful not to remove the flesh of the squash). Place cut-side down in the slow cooker.

Prepping

Pour the tomato sauce from the skillet into the slow cooker, over the squash. Arrange the meatballs in the sauce around the squash and make sure the meatballs are all covered in sauce. Cook on low for 7-8 hours or high for 3-4. Remove the spaghetti squash. Scoop out the spaghetti squash with fork and it will come apart in spaghetti-like strings. Portion into 6 glass containers and top with equal amounts of tomato sauce and meatballs. Top with parmesan. Refrigerate for up to 4 days and heat in the microwave.

Note: This is great when you're craving Italian food but don't want to spare the calories. Also this makes a great packable lunch for work too.

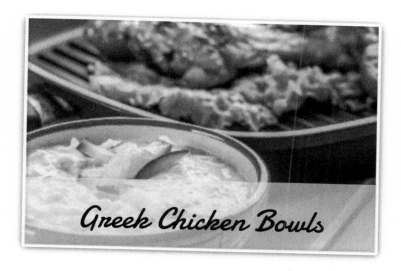

Greek Chicken Bowls

Serves 4 | Prep 30 min | Cook: 10 min | Ready in 1 HR

INGREDIENTS

1 lb boneless skinless chicken breast
¼ c. olive oil
2 tbsp. soy sauce
1/3 c. balsamic vinegar
1 tbsp. brown sugar
Black Pepper
Kosher Salt

For the Tzatziki:
1 cup Greek yogurt
½ cucumber, diced small
2 cloves garlic, minced very small
1 tablespoon lemon juice
1 teaspoon lemon zest plus
2 tablespoons chopped fresh dill
Kosher salt and freshly cracked black pepper

Bowls:
2 Cups Brown rice
1 firm tomato, diced
½ c. black olives sliced
¼ c. red onion, chopped

DIRECTIONS

1. Season the chicken breasts with salt and pepper.
2. In a small bowl whisk together oil, soy sauce, balsamic vinegar, and brown sugar. Place the chicken breasts in a ziplock bag and pour in the sauce. Squish around the chicken so its all evenly coated and place the bag in the fridge for at least 30 minutes.
3. Meanwhile, prepare the Tzatziki sauce: combine the yogurt, garlic, lemon juice, lemon zest, dill, and salt and pepper to taste. Set aside.
4. When the grill is nice and hot, place the chicken on the grill and grill for 3-4 minutes on each side or until the meat thermometer reads 165 degrees. Allow the chicken to sit for 5-10 minutes before cutting and serving.

PREPPING

In 4 glass containers, layer ½ cup brown rice, then ¼ of the chicken, dollop of tzatziki, then tomatoes, olives and onions. Refrigerate for up to 3 days.

Nutrition Per Serving:
Calories: 365, Fat: 18.5 g Carbs: 31.8, Fiber: 1.7 g, Protein: 18.8 g.

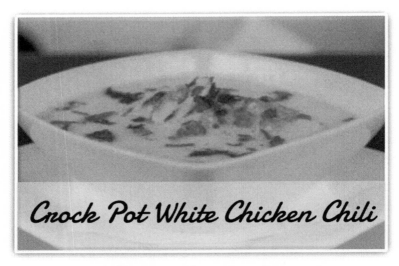

Crock Pot White Chicken Chili

Serves 4 | Prep 20 min | Cook: 7-8 hrs | Ready in 7-8 hrs

INGREDIENTS

1 1/2 lbs. Boneless, skinless chicken breasts or thighs
1 large yellow onion, diced
1 medium green bell pepper, chopped
1 small jalapeno, minced
4 cloves garlic, minced
3 tsp. ground cumin (add more to taste)
1 tsp. dried oregano
2 tsp. chili powder (add more to taste)
1 tsp. kosher salt
¼ tsp. black pepper
4 cups chicken stock
1 lime, juiced
½ cup fresh cilantro, chopped
½ cup chives chopped

DIRECTIONS

1. Throw the peppers, jalapeno, onion, garlic, spices into the slow cooker. Place the chicken on top and fill with all the broth.
2. Cook covered on low for 7-8 hours. Check the chicken with fork to see if it is falling apart.
3. Add the lime juice and stir, add salt and pepper to taste.

Prepping

When serving, top off with cilantro and chives. Store in the fridge for up to 5 days in glass. Heat in the microwave before eating.

Nutrition Per Serving:
Calories: **223**, Fat: 4.5 g Carbs: 9, Fiber: 2.3 g, Protein: 10 g.

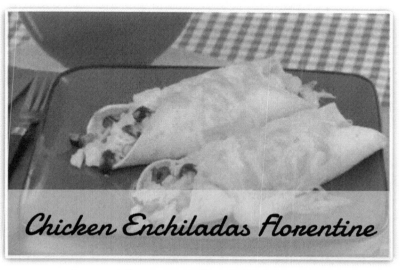

Chicken Enchiladas Florentine

Serves 4 | Prep 30 min | Cook: 30 Min | Ready in 1 HR

INGREDIENTS

1 lb. boneless skinless chicken breast, cooked and shredded
1 tablespoon olive oil
1 small yellow onion, diced
1 clove garlic, minced
4 cups fresh spinach leaves
1 tablespoon fresh lime juice
1/4 cup chopped cilantro
1/4 teaspoon ground cumin
1/4 teaspoon ground chili powder
Salt and black pepper, to taste
1 cup alfredo sauce, divided
½ c. water
4 burrito-sized tortillas
1 cup cheddar cheese

DIRECTIONS

1. In a large skillet, heat the olive oil over medium-high heat. Toss in onion, and garlic and stir sautéing until onions start to become translucent and garlic is fragrant.
2. Add in the spinach and lime and stir until the spinach is wilted and softens.
3. Add the cilantro, cumin, chili, salt and pepper. Then stir in ½ c. of alfredo sauce and stir until well combined, hot and bubbly. Mix in the shredded chicken

Prepping

Portion out the chicken spinach mixture into the four tortillas, roll them up and arrange them snugly in a square baking dish (lightly sprayed with cooking spray). Mix the other ½ cup of alfredo sauce with ½ cup of water. Pour the alfredo mixture evenly over the enchiladas. Sprinkle the cheese on top. Bake at 375 degrees F, for 20-30 minutes or until the cheese is melted and golden and the sauce is bubbly. Store directly in the glass baking pan covered with foil, and heat the leftovers in the microwave.

Nutrition Per Serving:

Calories: 404, Fat: 21.7 g Carbs: 28.5, Fiber: 2.1 g, Protein: 23.7 g.

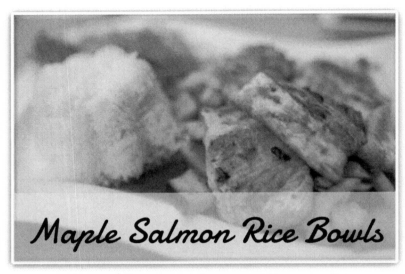

Maple Salmon Rice Bowls

Serves 4 | Prep 10 min | Cook: 10 min | Ready in 20 min

INGREDIENTS

4 (6 oz) wild salmon filets
1 1/2 tablespoon pure maple syrup
2 limes, juiced
1 teaspoon chili powder
3 cloves garlic, minced
1 tbsp. olive oil
1 1/2 cup brown rice, cooked
1 zucchini, diced
2 cups cauliflower florets
1 Avocado

DIRECTIONS

1. Whisk together the maple syrup, lime, chili, garlic.
2. Heat the olive oil in a large cast iron skillet. Toss in the chopped zucchini and cauliflower florets. Sear on all sides. As the vegetables start to soften, add in the salmon, and pour in the maple syrup mixture.
3. Sear salmon on both sides as sauce reduces. Cook to desired doneness.

PREPPING

To assemble the bowls (in 4 glass containers), scoop ¼th of the rice into a container, then add a salmon filet with one fourth of the vegetables and sauce, and top with sliced avocado. Refrigerate for up to 3 days.

Hint: don't add the avocado until just before eating so it doesn't turn brown.

NUTRITION PER SERVING:

Calories: 485, Fat: 23.4 g Carbs: 26.2, Fiber: 5.5 g, Protein: 43 g.

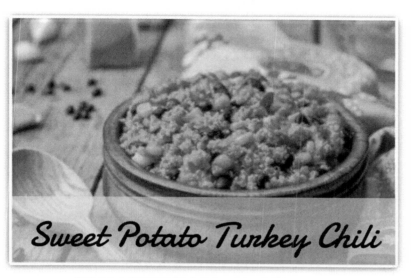

Sweet Potato Turkey Chili

Serves 6 | Prep 25 min | Cook: 3.5 HRS | Ready in 4 HRS

INGREDIENTS

1lb ground turkey
1 yellow onion, diced
4 cloves garlic, minced
¼ tsp. cayenne pepper (optional)
salt and pepper
3 cups chicken stock
2 (14.5 oz cans fire roasted tomatoes)
15 oz can black beans
1 cup sweet corn, from the can
1 cup dry quinoa
1 lb sweet potato, peeled and chopped into ½ inch cubes
2 Tablespoons chili powder
1 teaspoon cumin
1/2 teaspoon salt
¼ tsp. fresh black pepper
¼ c. fresh cilantro, chopped

DIRECTIONS

1. Brown the turkey, in a large skillet on the stop, then saute the onions in the meat juices until translucent. Add the garlic and continue stirring until fragrant and until the turkey is completely cooked (no pink visible). Add in the cayenne pepper and toss in a pinch of salt and pepper. Stir
2. Pour the meat mixture into the slow cooker and add all remaining ingredients except cilantro. Stir.

PREPPING

Cook on low for 3 to 3 and ½ hours or until potatoes are very tender. Or on low for 5-6 hours. Stir in Cilantro 15 minutes before eating. This one is great to throw together before leaving for work and set the timer on your slow cooker. Then you'll have a delicious meal waiting for you when you return. Portion the leftovers into glass meal prep containers and heat up in the microwave. This will keep for about 5 days in the fridge. You will have a delicious meal on Monday, and then lunch already packed for every day left in the week.

Nutrition Per Serving:

Calories: **409**, Fat: **4.6 g** Carbs: **59.8**, Fiber: **11.3 g**, Protein: **34.6 g.**

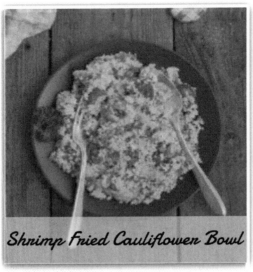

Shrimp Fried Cauliflower Bowl

Serves 4 | Prep 20 min | Cook: 0 | Ready in 20 min

INGREDIENTS

½ pound shrimp
1 teaspoon grated peeled fresh ginger
¼ teaspoon crushed red pepper
2 teaspoons dark sesame oil
1 red bell pepper
½ onion
Olive oil
1 clove garlic
4 cups cauliflower
1 egg
Cilantro (optional)

DIRECTIONS

1. Remove tails from the shrimp, chop the red pepper, onion, and garlic. Cut the cauliflower into very small pieces (or pulse lightly in the food processor). Combine the shrimp, chopped ginger, and crushed red pepper and toss until mixed.

2. Heat olive oil in your cast iron skillet. Add the chopped bell pepper, onion, and garlic and fry until cooked. Then add the shrimp mixture to pan and stir-fry until the shrimp isn't clear anymore. Add the chopped up cauliflower and sauté for another 2 minutes.

3. Crack an egg and whisk it in a separate bowl. Once whisked, toss it with shrimp and cauliflower, and stir-fry until egg is cooked.

4. Serve hot and garnish with fresh cilantro if desired.

Prepping

Refrigerate leftovers. If you prefer to have a fresh egg, repeat process until when it's time to add the egg, and only add it once it's time for you to eat. The best way to prepare the next few days when you're ready to eat is either microwave the rice in a dish with a little water, or heat it in a frying pan. Add some soy sauce and crack another egg into it. Eat as soon as its hot.

Note: you can just as easily use cooked brown rice for this dish, but please note the calorie content will be significantly higher.

Nutrition Per Serving:

Calories: 205, Fat: 11.5 g Carbs: 10.1, Fiber: 3.2 g, Protein: 16.8 g.

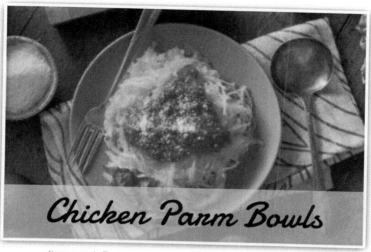

Chicken Parm Bowls

Serves 4 | Prep 40 min | Cook: 60 min | Ready in 1.6 Hrs

INGREDIENTS

2 tbsp. extra virgin olive oil
1 large Spaghetti Squash
2 c. Pomodoro sauce (plain marinara)
3 cloves garlic, minced
1 large yellow onion, diced
1 1/2 tsp. dried Italian seasoning
1 tsp. dried basil
Kosher salt and fresh black pepper to taste
1/4 tsp. fennel seeds (optional)
Red pepper flakes (optional)
1 lb boneless skinless chicken breast, cut into 4 equal pieces
2 tbsp flour
1 egg
¼ c. bran cereal, or low sodium bread crumbs
¼ c. finely grated parmesan

Prepping

In 4 microwave safe dishes, distribute the spaghetti squash evenly, then top with one of the chicken breasts, and finish with the rest of the tomato sauce. Top with more parmesan if desired. Heat in the microwave and store in the fridge for up to 3 days.

DIRECTIONS

1. In a skillet over medium heat, heat the olive oil. Sauté the onions for 5 minutes, then add the garlic and cook for 2 more minutes stirring. Make sure nothing is sticking to the bottom of the pan. Add the fire roasted tomatoes, the pomodoro and all the herbs and spices. Stir until everything is incorporated and reduce heat to medium low, leave for 15 minutes with the lid propped.
2. Slice the spaghetti squash in half, and scoop out the seeds and pulp. Brush lightly with olive oil and season with salt and pepper.
3. Place cut side down on a foil lined baking sheet and bake at 400 degrees F, for 40-50 minutes or until the squash is very tender.
4. While the squash is cooking, crack the egg into a flat shallow dish and add a few tbsp. of water beating the mixture until combined. In another flat shallow dish, mix together the bread crumbs and parmesan.
5. Take the 4 chicken pieces and very lightly sift the flour over them so they're even coated. Shake off the excess. Then dredge them in the egg mixture then in the parmesan bread crumb mixture evenly coating them.
6. In a large cast iron skillet, heat the other tablespoon of olive oil. Once the oil is hot, add the bread crumb coated chicken and sear until golden on both sides (2-3 min on each side).
7. Once you've seared the chicken, place in a square baking dish and pour a scoop of the tomato sauce mixture on each chicken piece. Bake in the oven (at the same time the squash is cooking) for about 20-25 minutes or until a meat thermometer reads 165 Degrees F.
8. When the squash is done, take a fork and scrape out all the flesh. It should break down into stringy, spaghetti-like pieces.

Nutrition Per Serving:

Calories: 332, Fat: 15.9 g Carbs: 30,
Fiber: 3.2 g, Protein: 20.9 g.

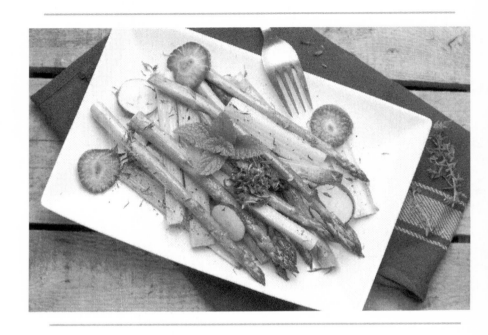

Cutting the Carbs

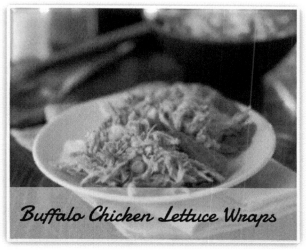

Buffalo Chicken Lettuce Wraps

Serves 4 | Prep 15min | Cook: 0-4HRS | Ready in 15 Min

INGREDIENTS

½ red pepper (diced)
½ green pepper (diced)
4 stalks of celery (diced)
2 lbs. of chicken thighs, skinless and boned, then chopped into bite sized pieced
2 scallions (sliced)
½ cup of crumbled blue cheese
2 tsp of onion powder, or a finely diced onion
1 tsp of garlic powder, or a crushed clove of garlic
2 tbsp. of butter
Salt and pepper to taste
Hot sauce to taste
8 large lettuce leaves (Bibb Lettuce works best)

DIRECTIONS

1. If you're using raw chicken breast, place the chicken into the slow cooker with the garlic, onion, chicken stock, and ranch seasoning and cook on low for 8 hours (or on high for 4 hours). If you are using canned chicken, just combine with garlic, onion, chicken stock, and ranch seasoning and cook for (1-2 hours)
2. 2. If you're not using the canned chicken, shred it with two forks. The canned chicken will already be shredded. Add the hot sauce, and the cream cheese and cheddar cheese. Combine and cook for 2 more hours on low (or one more hour on high).

Prepping

Store the buffalo chicken mixture in glass in the fridge for up to 5 days. Keep Lettuce leaves separate and don't assemble until you're ready to eat. If you're packing your lunch for work, just put the buffalo chicken mixture in a container in your lunch box and include the washed lettuce leaves wrapped in plastic separately.

Nutrition Per Serving:
Calories: 265, Fat: 16.2 g Carbs: 3.8, Fiber: 1 g, Protein: 25.5 g.

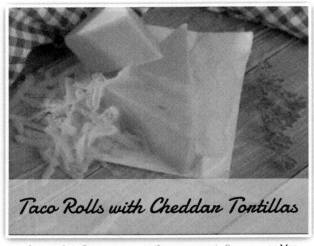

Taco Rolls with Cheddar Tortillas

Serves **6** | Prep **25** min | Cook: **15** min| Ready in **25** Min

INGREDIENTS

2 cups of cheddar cheese
1 cup of taco meat, left over or following the recipe below
¼ cup of tomatoes chopped
½ an avocado, chopped
2 tsp of taco sauce
Any other toppings you like, such as diced onions, olives and so on
1 lb. of ground or minced beef
1 tbsp. of chili powder
A clove of garlic, crushed
¼ of a small onion, diced very small
¼ tsp oregano
½ tsp paprika
Salt and pepper to taste

DIRECTIONS

1. Preheat the oven to 400 degrees.
2. Cover a baking tray with lightly greased grease proof paper or baking parchment, leaving some 'handles' to make it easy to lift.
3. Sprinkle the cheddar to make a single layer completely covering the tray. Grate more cheese if needed.
4. Cook for about 15 minutes until the cheese bubbles and browns.
5. While the cheese is cooking, combine the remaining ingredients. Remember that the layers will need to be not too chunky as you will be rolling the taco later.
6. Remove the cheese from the tray, using the parchment 'handles'.
7. Add the ingredients to the cheese mixture. Keep it to a single layer.
8. Roll it up from top to bottom, then once it's in roll form, slice it into rounds.

Prepping

wrap each roll in foil and store in the fridge. Unwrap and heat on a plate in the microwave. Top with a dollop of sour cream and your favorite salsa.

Nutrition Per Serving:

Calories: **284**, Fat: **18.9 g** Carbs: **3.4**, Fiber: **1.7 g**, Protein: **25 g**.

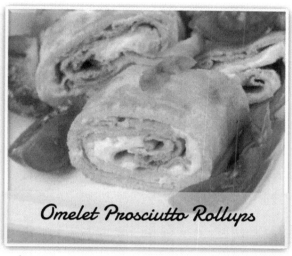

Omelet Prosciutto Rollups

Serves 4 | Prep 15 min | Cook: 5 min | Ready in 20 Min

INGREDIENTS

2 tbsp. Olive Oil

6 eggs

4 cups of spinach

6 slices, Prosciutto

6 oz goat cheese

¼ c. roasted red peppers (from jar) sliced thin

2 tbps fresh chives

Salt Pepper

DIRECTIONS

1. Whisk the eggs together vigorously for about 60 seconds. Add a few tbsp. of water, salt and pepper.
2. Heat 1 tbps oil in a large skillet over medium heat. Once the oil is hot, pour in 1/6 of the egg mixture. Swirl it aroun evenly and allow it to sit bubbling in the oil. Use a rubber spatula and continue to push the uncooked egg to the edges. Once the egg is no longer runny, turn the flat egg omelet onto a plate. Repeat this until you have 6 flat egg wraps.
3. In another tbsp. of oil, saute the spinach until wilted. Add salt and pepper to taste and stir in the roasted red peppers and chives.

Prepping

1. To assemble, place a slice of prosciutto on each egg wrap, then a scoop of the spinach mixture and then 1 oz of goat cheese. Roll the egg up and wrap it in waxed paper
2. Repeat for each rollup. Store in the fridge for up to 3 days, and heat in the microwave.

Note: serving size is 1 and a half rollups, but you can decide whatever you like for the serving size.

Nutrition Per Serving:

Calories: 362, Fat: 28.8 g Carbs: 4.5, Fiber: 1.1 g, Protein: 22.4 g.

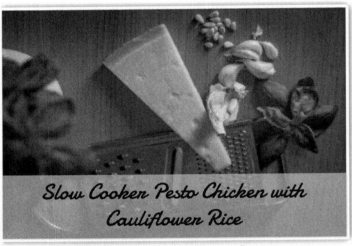

Slow Cooker Pesto Chicken with Cauliflower Rice

Serves 6 | Prep 25 min | Cook: 4-5 HRS | Ready in 4-5 HRS

INGREDIENTS

4 boneless skinless chicken breasts
1 c. pesto (either pre-made, or make your own using recipe provided)
1/2 c. water
1 large head of cauliflower
2 tsp. extra virgin olive oil
For the Pesto (makes more than a cup, store/freeze the excess):
3 cups packed fresh basil
3/4 cup grated Parmesan cheese
4 cloves garlic roughly chopped
1/2 cup extra virgin olive oil
1/4 cup pine nuts

Prepping

When the chicken is done, slice it up, and place pieces on a bed of the cauliflower rice. Spoon pesto sauce from the slow cooker over the chicken if desired. And portion out into 6 containers. Heat in a microwave. Store in the fridge for up to 3 days.

DIRECTIONS

1. To make the pesto, simply combine the basil, parmesan, garlic, olive oil and pine nuts into a blender or food processor and pulse until the entire mixture is smooth and combined. If you're using pre-made pesto, proceed to step 2.
2. In a medium bowl, whisk together 1 cup of pesto and the 1/2 cup of water until combined
3. Season the chicken breasts with salt and pepper and place in the slow cooker. Pour pesto mixture over the chicken
4. Cook for 4-5 hours on low, or 2-3 hours on high (or until chicken reads 165 degrees)
5. While the chicken is cooking, break the cauliflower into large sturdy chunks and grate it until the whole head has been grated.
6. Place grated cauliflower in a kitchen towel and wrap it tight and try to wring out any excess moisture from the cauliflower—try to get it as dry as you can. Pat with paper towels if necessary.
7. Heat 2 tsp. olive oil in a large skillet over medium heat. When the skillet is hot, add the cauliflower and stir so that it cooks evenly. Saute for 5-7 minutes until it's all cooked and tender.

Nutrition Per Serving:
Calories: 322, Fat: 22.7 g Carbs: 10.2, Fiber: 4.2 g, Protein: 20.9 g.

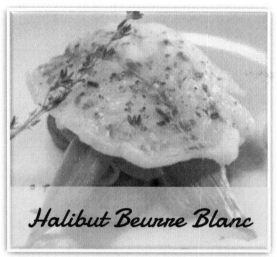

Halibut Beurre Blanc

Serves 6 | Prep 20 min | Cook: 10 min | Ready in 20 Min

INGREDIENTS

3 tablespoon extra-virgin olive oil

2 (8 ounce) halibut filets

1/2 cup white wine (chardonnay or equivalent)

2 teaspoon chopped garlic

2 Tablespoons of salted butter

½ tsp. kosher salt

¼ tsp. Cracked pepper

¼ cup capers

DIRECTIONS

1. Heat 2 tablespoons of olive oil in a skillet and pan fry the halibut searing on all sides until golden brown. Remove the fish from the pan and set on a plate.

2. Pour in the white wine and whisk making sure to scrape away any bits stuck on the bottom of the pan. Let the wine cook way down until all the alcohol has cooked off and you just have a small amount of liquid left and add the rest of the olive oil and all remaining ingredients and stir. Let it bubble up a bit then add the fish back to the pan and cook basting with the sauce until the fish is fully cooked and flakey.

3. Serve and pour the residual sauce over the fish and serve with lemon wedge and fresh dill sprig if desired. Serve with fresh vegetables of your choice

Prepping

you can make the wine sauce ahead and store in a glass jar, but you'll want to fry up the fish the day of. Keep the ingredients on hand and throw it together in a few minutes before eating. I love to fry up the fish with some fresh veggie slike bok choy and carrots, or asparagus and Brussel sprouts. It makes for a really quick meal if you have the ingredients on hand and have the wine sauce ready to go.

Nutrition Per Serving:
Calories: 259, Fat: 16.8 g Carbs: 1.7, Fiber: 0.3 g, Protein: 20.4 g.

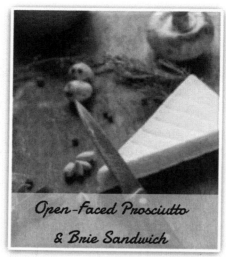

Open-Faced Prosciutto

& Brie Sandwich

SERVES 4 | PREP 10min | COOK: 0 HRS | READY in 10 Min

INGREDIENTS

2 avocados
4 small slices of brie
8 thin slices of prosciutto
10 mushrooms (any variety, but large flat ones work well)
2 cup of raw spinach
2 tsp of butter
Pinch salt
A sprinkle of black pepper

DIRECTIONS

1. Cook the spinach for five minutes until it has wilted. Drain and squeeze out excess water.
2. Slice the mushroom and sauté in the butter until soft. Add some pepper and salt.
3. Cut the avocado in half. Do this by cutting until the pit is reached, then rotating and twisting until the avocado splits. Remove the stone and scoop out the flesh. Cut a slice off the bottom of one half of the avocado so it can stand. This will be your 'bottom slice of bread'.
4. Fill the two halves of your avocado with the ingredients. Serve as open-faced sandwich

PREPPING

Wrap the stuffed avocado halves in plastic and squirt with fresh lemon or lime and store in the fridge. Heat in the microwave. I like to top mine with a fried egg.

NUTRITION PER SERVING:

Calories: 310, Fat: 24.5 g Carbs: 5.4, Fiber: 3.5 g, Protein: 20 g.

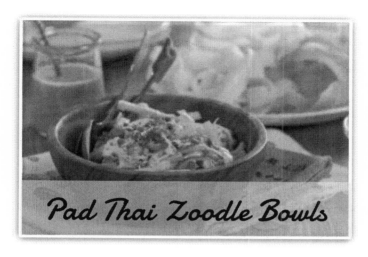

Pad Thai Zoodle Bowls

Serves 4 | Prep 20min | Cook: 10 min | Ready in 30 Min

INGREDIENTS

1 tbsp. olive oil
½ lb. chicken breast, chopped
2 large zucchinis, spiralized
2-3 scallions, sliced
1/4 cup chopped peanuts
1/3 cup finely chopped cilantro
½ cup bean sprouts
½ c. chopped scallions
2 eggs

Sauce
2 tbsp low-sodium soy sauce
1 tbsp peanut butter
2 cloves garlic minced
2 tbsp fish sauce
1 tbsp lime juice
1 tbsp. brown sugar

DIRECTIONS

1. Spiral the zucchinis or chop them into matchsticks.
2. Whisk together the ingredients for the sauce.
3. Heat the oil in a large skillet, and add the chicken. Add half the sauce. Stir and cook until chicken is fully cooked (about 10 minutes).
4. Toss in the zucchini noodles and saute until the noodles are tender (about1 minutes). Crack in the two eggs. And mix around until the eggs are fully cooked and evenly distributed.
5. Remove from heat and portion out into meal prep containers.

PREPPING
Portion out the Pad Thai into Meal Prep containers and top with Scallions, Bean Sprouts and lime wedge. Store in the fridge for up to 3 days. To reheat, simply remove the lime wedge and heat in the microwave, then squirt on the lime juice and enjoy!

Nutrition Per Serving:

Calories: 255, Fat: 14.1 g Carbs: 13.3, Fiber: 3.2 g, Protein: 22.4 g.

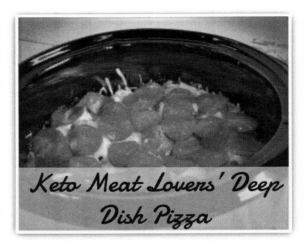

Keto Meat Lovers' Deep Dish Pizza

Serves 6 | Prep 20 min | Cook: 2 HRS | Ready in: 2.5 HRS

INGREDIENTS

1 lb. lean ground beef, browned and drained and seasoned with salt and pepper
Kosher salt
Fresh ground black pepper
1 lb. lean ground turkey
1/4 tsp. fennel seeds
1/2 tsp. Italian Seasoning
1/2 tsp. dried oregano
1/2 tsp garlic powder
6 strips of bacon, fried and crumbled
2 oz. turkey pepperoni
1 (14-oz) jar pizza sauce
1 large green pepper
1 medium onion
1 (6oz) package mushrooms, chopped
1 c. mozzarella cheese
5 slices provolone cheese

DIRECTIONS

1. Brown the ground turkey over medium heat in a large skillet, draining as necessary. While the meat is browning, add the fennel, Italian seasoning, and garlic powder. Break the meat down until crumbly. Add the green pepper and onion and mushrooms and continue to cook until vegetables start to soften (about 5 minutes). Season with salt and pepper.
2. Pour 1/2 c. pizza sauce into the bottom of the slow cooker, then spread the browned ground beef over the bottom. Pour 1/2 c. of the sauce over that layer and spread. Layer the provolone for the next layer. Then add the ground turkey and vegetables and spread. Pour rest of pizza sauce over the ground turkey layer, then spread the pepperoni and bacon across that layer. Top with the mozzarella.
3. Cook on low for 2 hours. (for Vegetarian options, you can substitute egg and zucchini and eggplant for the meat)

Prepping

store in the fridge directly in the glass slow cooker pan. Slice into pie slices and heat in the microwave before eating. Store covered for up to 3 days.

Nutrition Per Serving:

Calories: 429, Fat: 22.1 g Carbs: 11.9, Fiber: 2.1 g, Protein: 44.9 g.

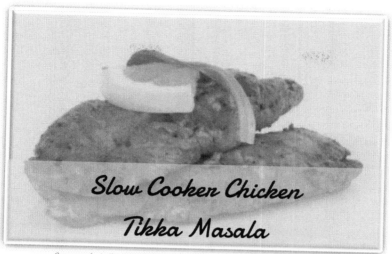

Slow Cooker Chicken Tikka Masala

Serves **6** | Prep **35 min** | Cook: **4-6 HRS** | Ready in: **4-6 HRS**

INGREDIENTS

6 medium (boneless, skinless), cut into 1-inch cubes
1 tablespoons vegetable oil
1 tbsp. butter
2 medium onions, chopped
3 cloves garlic, minced
1 tbsp. madras paste
3 tsp. madras powder
1 tsp. garam masala
1 inch ginger root, minced (about 1tbsp.)
1/2 tsp. ground cumin
1/4 tsp. nutmeg
1/3 c. tomato paste
1 c. crushed tomatoes
1c. tomato puree
1/2 c. coconut milk
1 c. Greek yogurt (plain, unsweetened)

DIRECTIONS

1. In a large skillet, heat oil and butter on medium-high heat until the butter is melted and the mixture is combined. Add the onions and sauté for about 3-5 minutes until onions start to become translucent. Add the minced garlic and stir for about 30 seconds, then add the chicken breasts and sear on both sides (about 2-3 minutes on each side).
2. Turn off the heat and add all remaining ingredients stirring until totally combined.
3. Pour the mixture into the slowcooker.
4. Cook on high for 4-6 hours, or low for 7-8 hours. Garnish with chopped scallions (if desired) and serve with a lemon wedge.

Prepping

store in glass in the fridge for up to 4 days. Heat in the microwave and serve with fresh lemon.

Nutrition Per Serving:

Calories: **298**, Fat: **12.7 g** Carbs: **16.3**, Fiber: **4 g**, Protein: **30.5 g**.

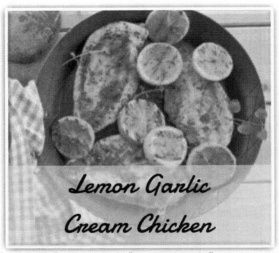

Lemon Garlic Cream Chicken

Serves 4 | Prep 30 min | Cook: 10 mins | Ready in: 40 min

INGREDIENTS

4 boneless skinless chicken breasts
2 tablespoons lemon juice
6 cloves minced garlic
2 tablespoons fresh basil, chopped
½ tsp. Italian Seasoning
1 cup chicken stock
Salt and pepper
1 tablespoon olive oil
1 small yellow onion
2 tablespoons salted butter
¼ cup heavy cream

DIRECTIONS

1. Mix together the chicken stock, lemon and garlic basil and Italian seasoning.
2. Heat the oil in a large cast iron skillet (or any oven-safe skillet). Saute the onions until translucent, then add the chicken breasts. Sear for 2-3 minutes on both sides. Remove the chicken and put on a plate
3. Add in the chicken broth mixture to the onions, and whisk simmering the sauce until it reduces.
4. Then stir in the butter until melted and well combined. Remove the skillet from the heat and stir in the heavy cream. Place back on the heat (on low) stirring just until the sauce is hot again. Do not allow it to boil or else the cream may scorch or curdle).
5. Add the chicken back into the pan and toss it until completely coated in the sauce.
6. Place the cast iron in the oven baking at 350 degrees for 7-10 minutes or until the chicken is fully cooked and a meat thermometer reads 165 degrees F.

Prepping

Portion the chicken into 4 microwave safe dishes and top with a fresh lemon wedge. Store in the fridge for up to 3 days. To heat, simply remove the lemon wedge, microwave, then squirt on the fresh lemon and enjoy! Serve with a green salad or steamed veggies for a super easy meal.

Nutrition Per Serving:

Calories: 247, Fat: 14 g Carbs: 3.8, Fiber: 0.5 g, Protein: 27 g.

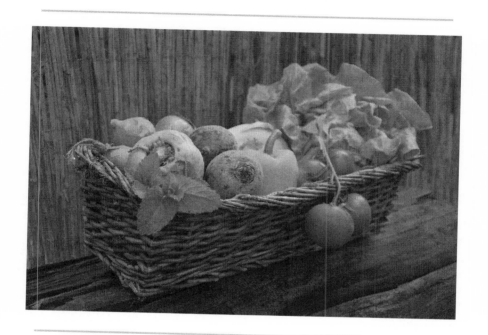

Vegetarian Dishes

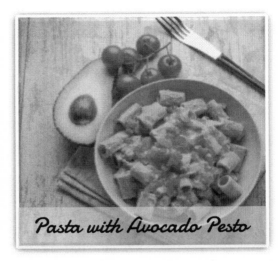

Pasta with Avocado Pesto

Serves 4 | Prep 15 min | Cook: 15 mins | Ready in: 30 min

INGREDIENTS

Pesto:
1 avocado fully ripe, peeled and pitted, roughly diced
2 cups of fresh basil
1/2 cup of walnuts
6 peeled cloves of garlic
A Few tbsp. water
1 lemon
1/2 cup of grated Parmesan cheese
2 tbsp of olive oil
Salt and pepper to taste

Pasta
½ c. Grape Tomatoes, diced
1 lb of pasta of choice (I choose spinach rigatoni, but you can use whole wheat or vegetable pasta, or to cut calories, use Zucchini Noodles or Spaghetti Squash)

DIRECTIONS

1. In a food processor, combine all the pesto ingredients and pulse until smooth. Add water little by little until it reaches the desired consistency. Taste it and season with salt and pepper to your liking.
2. Prepare the Pasta according to the package directions. Then drain and allow the pasta to cool slightly.

Prepping

Toss the pasta in the Avocado pesto. Portion into glass meal prep containers and squeeze extra lemon on top to keep avocado from turning brown. Heat in the microwave before eating. Store in the fridge for up to 3 days.

Nutrition Per Serving:
Calories: 313, Fat: 19.8 g Carbs: 25.3, Fiber: 5.9 g, Protein: 14 g.

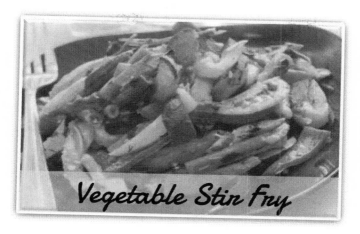

Vegetable Stir Fry

SERVES 4 | PREP 20 min | COOK: 10 mins | READY in: 30 min

INGREDIENTS

8 oz tofu or tempeh
2 tbsp. Olive oil
1 large zucchini
1 large eggplant
1 (6oz) container mushrooms
2 Medium carrots
2 Large Onions
1 Red Bell Pepper
1 Green Bell Pepper
6 cloves garlic, minced
2 tbsp fresh ginger, minced
1 red chili pepper, minced
¼ c. low sodium soy sauce
¼ tsp. black pepper
Lime

DIRECTIONS

1. Wash, and prepare all vegetables for the stir fry.
2. Heat 1 tbsp olive oil in a large cast iron. Toss in the tofu cubes once the pan is nice and hot. Sear the tofu on all sides. Then Remove from the pan.
3. Drizzle in the other tablespoon of olive oil and add all the vegetables. Once the vegetables start to soften and the garlic becomes fragrant, add in the soy sauce and pepper.

PREPPING

Store in a large glass container and serve over rice or in a wrap. To reheat, I heat in a nonstick skillet, but you can also use the microwave.

NUTRITION PER SERVING:
Calories: 234, Fat: 10.2 g Carbs: 30.7, Fiber: 9.5 g, Protein: 10.6 g.

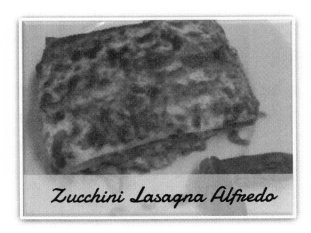

Zucchini Lasagna Alfredo

Serves 6 | Prep 30 min | Cook: 2-3 HRS | Ready in: 2.5-3.5 HRS

INGREDIENTS

3 medium zucchini
2tsp. extra virgin olive oil
2 c. Prepared Alfredo sauce
1/2 tsp. Italian seasoning
1 tbsp. fresh basil
2 cloves garlic, minced
Kosher salt
Fresh ground black pepper
16 ounces low-fat ricotta
1 (10oz) package frozen spinach, thawed and drained
2 large eggs
1 tsp garlic powder
1/3 c. grated parmesan
6 slices provolone cheese
Fresh Parsley

PREPPING

Set your slow cooker on auto timer and then throw the dish together and get on with your day. (Great for a Saturday or Sunday). Then Store the lasagna in the slow cooker pan, covered in the fridge for up to 5 days. Scoop out one portion at a time and heat in the microwave, or scoop into your meal prep glass containers and pack your lunches for work.

DIRECTIONS

1. Slice the zucchini as thin as possible—about ¼ inch. (use a mandoline if you have one), then place the zucchini strips on baking sheets and broil on high for about 8 minutes turning once. You may need to lightly spray the zucchini with cooking spray. Remove the broiled zucchini from the oven, drain off any excess liquid and set aside

2. In a skillet, heat the olive oil and sauté the garlic for 2 minutes over medium heat. Add the alfredo sauce Italian seasoning and fresh basil. Season with salt and pepper to taste. Set aside.

3. Drain the ricotta of excess liquid, then combine in a mixing bowl with the drained thawed spinach, the eggs, garlic powder, and grated parmesan. Mix together until all ingredients are thoroughly combined.

4. Spoon a few scoops of alfredo sauce into the bottom of the slow cooker. Then layer the first layer of broiled zucchini in the slow cooker, follow with 1/3 of the ricotta mixture, then 1/3 of the alfredo sauce.

5. Cook on high for 2-3 hours, or low for 4-5. 30 minutes before serving, layer the provolone on top of the lasagna. Continue to cook until the cheese is melted.

6. Garnish with fresh parsley and serve

Nutrition Per Serving:

Calories: 347, Fat: 23.2 g Carbs: 12, Fiber: 2.2 g, Protein: 25 g.

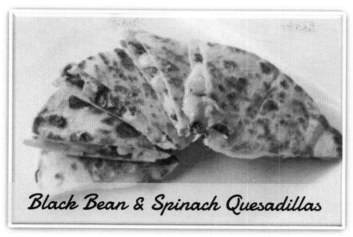

Black Bean & Spinach Quesadillas

Serves **6** | Prep **15 min** | Cook: **10 min** | Ready in: **20-25 min**

INGREDIENTS

19 oz can of black or white beans
3 cups fresh spinach
1 teaspoon ground cumin
2 tbps. Fresh cilantro, chopped
½ tsp. garlic powder
1/8 teaspoon salt
2 cups shredded mozzarella or provolone cheese
6 large tortillas

DIRECTIONS

1. In a medium bowl, smash the black beans with a fork and add the spinach, cilantro, cumin, garlic powder and salt. Continue mashing until the spinach wilts a bit.
2. Spray a non stick skillet with cooking spray and make the quesadillas by putting the tortilla in the pan, and spreading about 1/3 cup of the black bean mixture, and then 1/3 cup of shredded cheese. Fold over the tortilla in half.
3. Cook over medium heat slowly so the tortilla doesn't burn, but everything cooks inside. About 4 minutes on each side. Repeat for the rest of the tortillas. (you should be able to do 2 at a time once you fold them in half

PREPPING

Wrap the tortillas in waxed paper and heat in the microwave before eating. They also freeze well, so you can wrap them in waxed paper and then put them all in a large freezer bag and simply pop them in the microwave as needed.

NUTRITION PER SERVING:
Calories: **281**, Fat: **14.1 g** Carbs: **22.6**, Fiber: **2.8 g**, Protein: **16.2 g**.

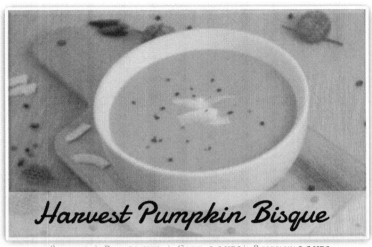

Harvest Pumpkin Bisque

Serves 5 | Prep 20 min | Cook: 2-5 HRS | Ready in: 2-5 HRS

INGREDIENTS

1 Medium pumpkin (butternut, sugar etc) (if using canned, about 3-1/2 cups canned pumpkin)
1 medium swt. potato, peeled and diced
2 carrots, chopped
1 medium yellow onion, chopped
2 c. vegetable stock
1 tsp. curry powder
½ tsp. ground ginger
½ tsp. ground nutmeg
½ tsp. cumin
1 c. heavy cream
Kosher salt
Freshly ground black pepper
Low fat sour cream (optional)

DIRECTIONS

1. Peel pumpkin skin, and remove pulp and seeds (save seeds if desired). Cube up the pumpkin flesh.
2. Place pumpkin, potato, carrots, onion, vegetable stock, and spices in the slow cooker.
3. Cook on low for 4-5 hours or high for 2-3. Make sure vegetables are extremely tender.
4. Pour contents of the slow cooker into a blender and pulse until the vegetables are completely broken down and the mixture is smooth and even.
5. Pour the mixture back into the slow cooker and add in the heavy cream stirring until thoroughly mixed. Season with salt and pepper as desired. Heat back up to desired heat and serve.
6. Serve garnished with a dollop of sour cream and toasted pumpkin seeds if desired.

PREPPING

Store in a glass container in the fridge for up to 5 or 6 days. Simply heat in the microwave before consuming. This goes great with a hearty wholegrain bread and a light green salad

Nutrition Per Serving:

Calories: 195, Fat: 9.6 g Carbs: 27, Fiber: 7.3 g, Protein: 3.4 g.

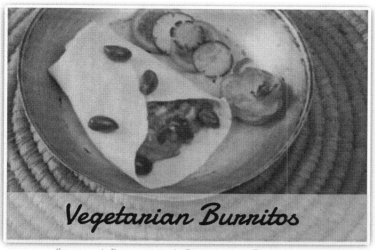

Vegetarian Burritos

Serves 4 | Prep 30 min | Cook: 0 HRS | Ready in: 30 min

INGREDIENTS

½ tbps. Olive oil
2 cups black beans,
4 eggs
1 (14.5 oz) can fire-roasted tomatoes
1 summer squash, chopped into half moons
1 zucchini chopped into half moons.
1 large yellow onion, chopped
1 red bell pepper
1 Green Bell Pepper
1 jalapeno
¼ c. chopped cilantro
3 tbsp low sodium taco seasoning
4 Tortillas (whole wheat recommended)
1 cup mozzarella cheese

DIRECTIONS

1. Drain and rinse the black beans, and beat the eggs in a small bowl.
2. In a large skillet, coat with cooking spray, and pour in the beans and stir in the taco seasoning and the can of stewed tomatoes. Add a few tbsp of water and let the mixture simmer until the water has mostly cooked off. Pour in the beaten eggs. As they start to scramble, stir until eggs are fully cooked. Remove from the pan and pour into a large bowl.
3. In the skillet, heat the olive oil. Once the oil is hot, add the onions, peppers and jalapeno. After about 2 minutes of sautéing, add the zucchini and summer squash. Continue sautéing until the vegetables are all tender and slightly caramelized.

Prepping

To assemble the burritos, scoop ¼ of the egg/bean mixture into the burrito, then ¼ of the veggies, then sprinkle on some fresh cilantro, and finally, top with ¼ c. of cheese. Roll the burrito up and wrap it in foil. Store in the fridge for up to 4 days. When you're ready to eat, simply remove the foil and microwave until the burrito is hot and the cheese is melted.

Nutrition Per Serving:

Calories: 279, Fat: 9.5 g Carbs: 36.1, Fiber: 8.8 g, Protein: 15.3 g.

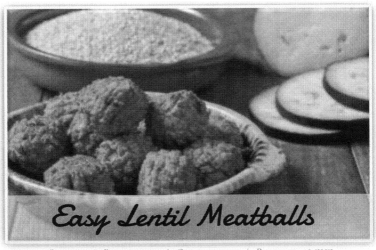
Easy Lentil Meatballs

Serves 4 | Prep 30 min | Cook: 10 min | Ready in: 40 min

INGREDIENTS

1 tbps. Olive oil
1 small yellow onion, diced
1 cup dried lentils
1 1/2 cups vegetable stock
3 cloves garlic, minced
1/2 cup panko bread crumbs
1/2 cup freshly grated parmesan cheese
1/4 cup chopped fresh Italian parsley
1 1/2 tablespoons tomato paste
1 teaspoon dried Italian seasoning
1/2 teaspoon kosher salt
1/4 teaspoon black pepper
2 large eggs

DIRECTIONS

1. Cook lentils according to package instructions in the vegetable stock.
2. Meanwhile, heat oil in a skillet and sauté the onions until they're translucent (about 4 minutes) on medium heat. Add the garlic, and stir. Cook for another 60 seconds then remove from heat.
3. Put the lentils in the food processor and pulse until they're broken down but slightly coarse. In a bowl, mix together all the ingredients. Once the mixture is completely mixed the texture should be moist enough to roll into balls, but not too wet to do so, roll into balls (about the size of a golf ball)
4. Place on a greased cookie sheet and bake at 425 for about 10 minutes or until the balls are golden and slightly crispy on the outside but still moist inside.

Prepping

You can freeze these, or store them in the fridge for up to 5 days. Heat in the microwave or on the stope top with your favorite sauce: (alfredo, pesto, marinara etc), serve over pasta or rice. (to cut calories even more, serve over zucchini noodles or spaghetti squash or cauliflower rice).

Note: the serving size is 3-4 meatballs, depending on the size you make them.

Nutrition Per Serving:

Calories: 266, Fat: 9.1 g Carbs: 29.2, Fiber: 10.7 g, Protein: 18 g.

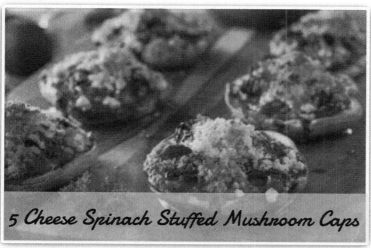

5 Cheese Spinach Stuffed Mushroom Caps

Serves 6 | Prep 20 min | Cook: 20 min | Ready in: 40 min

INGREDIENTS

1.5 lbs Portobello mushrooms
10 oz fresh spinach
¼ cup ricotta
½ cup parmesan, grated
¼ cup cheddar cheese, grated
3.5 oz goat cheese
1 cup cream cheese (Use Neufchatel Cheese, it's lower cal)
2 tbsp butter
1/8 tsp dried Italian herbs
2 tbsp red bell pepper, diced
½ small red onion, chopped
½ tsp garlic, minced

PREPPING

Wrap the mushroom caps in plastic and store in the fridge for up to 3 days, only cook right before eating. When youre ready to eat, remove the plastic wrap and lace the baking tray in the oven for 20 minutes. The mushroom topping should turn slightly brown and appear bubbly. Garnish with some fresh herbs and serve. If anything is left over, you can use it as stuffing for chicken breasts.

DIRECTIONS

1. Preheat the oven to 355 degrees F.
2. Remove the stems and gills of the mushrooms. Use a paper towel to thoroughly dry the mushroom caps.
3. Melt the butter in a pan and pour in a small bowl. Use a brush to smear the melted butter over the mushroom caps. Make sure you brush both the inside and outside.
4. Line a baking tray with parchment paper and place the mushroom caps on the tray.
5. Finely chop the spinach leaves and red onion. Place them in a large bowl and add the ricotta, parmesan, cream cheese, goat cheese, and minced garlic. Mix the ingredients well.
6. Use a spoon to scoop the mixture into the mushroom caps. Don't be afraid to fill the mushroom caps all the way to the top and then some. The mixture will not melt and run in the oven.
7.Top the mixture with the diced red peppers and grated cheddar cheese.

Nutrition Per Serving:

Calories: 323, Fat: 24.8 g Carbs: 9.5, Fiber: 2.3 g, Protein: 18.9 g.

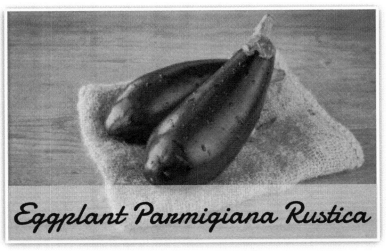

Eggplant Parmigiana Rustica

Serves 6 | Prep 30 min | Cook: 4-5 HRS | Ready in: 4.5-5.5 HRS

INGREDIENTS

2 tbsp. extra virgin olive oil, divided
2 large eggplants, sliced in rounds
(about ½ inch thick)
2 eggs
1/2 c. grated parmesan cheese (use
the type that is dry and powdery
that comes in a can)
2 c. Pomodoro (plain marinara)
3 cloves of garlic, minced
1 large yellow onion, diced
1 tsp. Italian seasoning
1/2 tsp. kosher salt
1/4 tsp. fresh ground black pepper
12 slices of provolone cheese
Fresh grated Parmesan

Prepping

Store in a glass baking dish
wrapped in foil, and scoop out
one servings at a time and
microwave until hot.

DIRECTIONS

1. Brush each of the eggplant rounds lightly with 1 tbsp.
olive oil and season with salt and pepper. Set aside.
2. Heat remaining tbsp. olive oil in a skillet and saute the
onions at medium heat until translucent and softening (5-7
minutes). Add garlic and continue cooking for 2 minutes
stirring. Add the Pomodoro, Italian seasoning, salt and
pepper. Pour a few scoops of the sauce into the bottom of
the slow cooker and set the rest aside.
3. Whisk the eggs together (add water if necessary) and
pour into shallow flat bowl. Take another shallow flat bowl
and pour in 1/2c. parmesan. Take each eggplant round and
dip it into the egg wash coating all sides, and then dredge it
briefly in the parmesan shaking off the excess. Layer the
battered eggplant in the slow cooker. When you have one
layer completed, top each eggplant round with a slice of
provolone. Spoon some tomato sauce on and spread it
around and then start the next layer.
4. When the eggplant layers are finished, pour the rest of
the tomato sauce over the eggplant into the slow cooker.
5. Cook on high for 4-5 hours or low for 8 hours
6. Serve with fresh grated parmesan cheese if desired and
garnish with fresh basil.

Nutrition Per Serving:

Calories: 414, Fat: 26.8 g Carbs: 21.4,
Fiber: 8.1 g, Protein: 25.1 g.

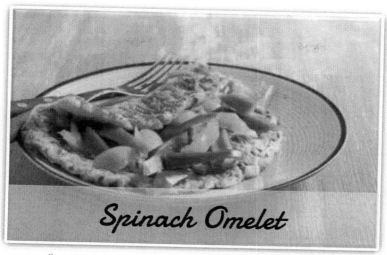

Spinach Omelet

Serves 4 | Prep 10 min | Cook: 10 min | Ready in: 20 min

INGREDIENTS

6 large eggs
3 oz feta cheese, crumbled
2 tbps. Olive oil
6 oz spinach
2 cloves garlic
1 red bell pepper
1 yellow bell pepper
Salt and pepper, to taste

Prepping

Wrap each omelet in plastic wrap and store in the fridge for up to 3 days. Heat in the microwave before eating.

DIRECTIONS

1. Heat pan with one tablespoon of Olive oil. Slice the garlic and cook over medium-high heat. Add salt and cook for one minute.
2. Cook the spinach leaves in the pan for two minutes and then pour the spinach and garlic into a bowl.
3. Take a small bowl and crack the eggs into it. Beat with a fork and add the spinach and crumbled feta. Season with salt and pepper.
4. Grease the pan with the remaining ghee and cook the mixture over medium heat. Move the egg mixture toward the middle of the pan using a spatula for 30 seconds. Reduce heat and cook for one minute. Take your time when cooking to produce a fluffy and soft omelet.
5. Slice the green and yellow bell peppers and use as topping on the omelet.
6. Fold up the omelet and cook for one minute to warm the peppers. Repeat for the other 3 omelets.

Nutrition Per Serving:

Calories: 254, Fat: 19.3 g Carbs: 8, Fiber: 1.8 g, Protein: 14.4 g.

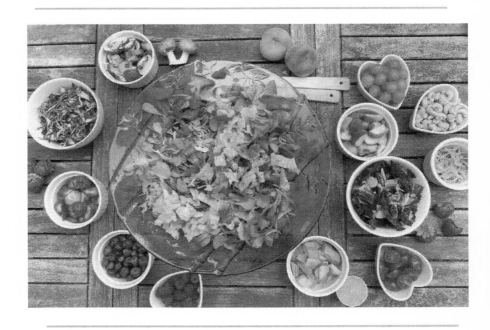

Plant-Based Meals

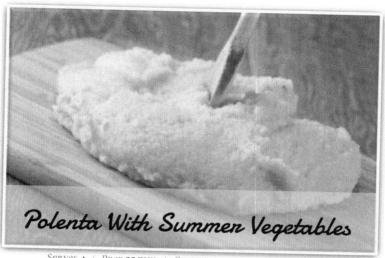

Polenta With Summer Vegetables

Serves 4 | Prep 25 min | Cook: 15 min | Ready in: 40 min

INGREDIENTS

2 tablespoons olive oil
1 bell pepper, seeded and chopped
1 eggplant, diced into small pieces
1 large zucchini, diced into small pieces
6 cups water
1 1/2 dry polenta
1/4 teaspoon cracked black pepper
10 ounces frozen spinach, thawed and drained
½ cup cherry tomatoes, halved
¼ cup kalamata olives, chopped
1 tsp. dried Italian seasoning

DIRECTIONS

1. Toss the eggplant zucchini and peppers in one tbsp. of olive oil and spread over a cookie sheet. Place under the broiler on low in the center rack. When the vegetables start to caramelize and become tender remove from the oven.
2. In a medium pot, boil the water and stir in the dry polenta. Cook and stir as it thickens for about 5 minutes. Once the mixture gets thick and custardy, stir in the butter and black pepper.
3. Spread the polenta batter into a greased square baking pan and brush the top with olive oil. Bake at 350 for about 10 minutes.
4. Top with spinach and then add the tomatoes and olives, and next the roasted vegetables and finally the Italian seasoning. Add kosher salt to taste. Bake for 10 more minutes, and then slice into wedges and serve.

PREPPING

Wrap each omelet in plastic wrap and store in the fridge for up to 3 days. Heat in the microwave before eating.

NUTRITION PER SERVING:

Calories: 214, Fat: 9.2 g Carbs: 30.9, Fiber: 8 g, Protein: 6.1 g.

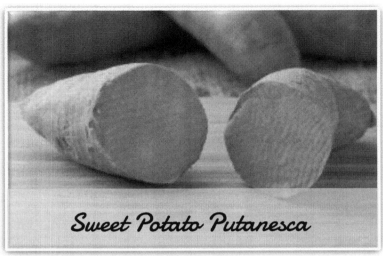

Sweet Potato Putanesca

Serves 6 | Prep 25 min | Cook: 15 min | Ready in: 40 min

INGREDIENTS

Olive oil
6 garlic cloves
2 teaspoons dried oregano
1 teaspoon crushed red pepper
2 cups unsalted chicken stock
6 cups sweet potatoes
6 cups cherry tomatoes
2 tablespoons unsalted tomato paste
¼ cup chopped fresh basil
¼ cup chopped fresh parsley
½ cup black olives
3 tablespoons capers

DIRECTIONS

1. Mince the garlic and cut the sweet potato into French fry like pieces. Chop the cherry tomatoes into two or three pieces each. Do the same for the black olives.
2. Add olive oil the cast iron skillet and bring stove to a medium heat. Add the garlic, cut anchovies, dried oregano, and peppers to the skillet and cook for a few minutes while tossing the food. Then add stock and bring to a boil.
3. Once the food is boiling, add the sweet potato slices, tomatoes, along with the tomato paste. Cook until the sweet potato is softened. Then add the olives and capers.

Prepping

Serve with fresh basil and parsley. Refrigerate leftovers, but keep the basil and parsley separate from the rest of the food to preserve their freshness. Keep in glass 3-4 days. You can microwave to heat and eat.

Nutrition Per Serving:

Calories: 344, Fat: 7.9 g Carbs: 53.7, Fiber: 9.9 g, Protein: 16.3 g.

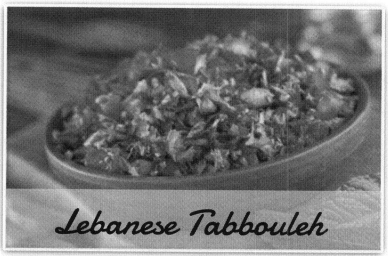

Lebanese Tabbouleh

SERVES 4 | PREP 15 min | COOK: 0 min | READY in: 15 min

INGREDIENTS

1 cup firm tomatoes, chopped small
1/2 cup bulgur wheat
1 medium cucumber, diced small
2 cups loosely packed Italian Parsley, stems removed, chopped
1/4 cup chopped fresh mint
1/3 cup green onion, chopped small
Kosher salt and black pepper
¼ c. freshly squeezed Lemon Juice
¼ c. Extra virgin Olive Oil
Baby Spinach (optional)

DIRECTIONS

1. Put the bulgar wheat in a small bowl and cover with water. Soak for 5-6 minutes, drain off the water, and put the wheat in a kitchen towel and squeeze out any excess water
2. Combine all ingredients in a large bowl mixing well and seasoning with salt and pepper to taste. Allow to chill at least 30 minutes before serving. (Note: make sure the vegetables and herbs are chopped very fine for best results).

PREPPING

you can reserve the lemon juice and oil until the day of consumption. Without the oil and lemon, you can store the salad in glass for up to 3 days in the fridge. Add the oil and lemon and mix well before eating.

NUTRITION PER SERVING:

Calories: 207, Fat: 13.4 g Carbs: 21.1, Fiber: 5.8 g, Protein: 2.3 g.

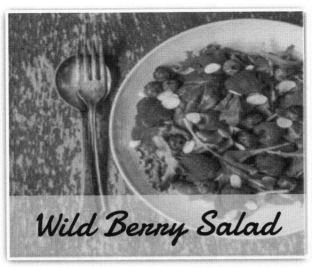

Wild Berry Salad

Serves 6 | Prep 15 min | Cook: 0 min | Ready in: 15 min

INGREDIENTS

1 cup chickpeas
Oregano
1/2 cup blueberries
1/2 cup raspberries
¼ cup slivered toasted almonds
10 Roma tomatoes
3 cups baby spinach

Dressing:
1/4 c. balsamic vinegar
1/4 c. olive oil
1 tsp. Dried Italian Seasoning
½ tsp. Garlic Powder
¼ tsp. Salt
¼ tsp. Black Pepper

DIRECTIONS

1. Whisk together all the ingredients for the dressing
2. Take 5 Mason Jars and pour 3 tablespoons of olive oil into each. Then add as much vinegar as you like for the dressing.
3. Sprinkle fresh oregano on the dressing. Cut tomatoes and place them on top of the dressing. Use two tomatoes per jar (10 total). Divide them equally and put them into each Mason jar. Crush goat cheese and add equal portions to the salads as well.
4. Divide the blueberries into five equal portions and add them to the salads. Finally, place the spinach on top and close the Mason Jar.

PREPPING

Refrigerate for the entire workweek. When it is time to eat the salads, shake them in the Mason jar first to mix the densest material (dressing) with the rest of the salad. Make sure to only mix right before consumption, or the salad will get wet and rot quicker.

Nutrition Per Serving:

Calories: 364, Fat: 19.3 g Carbs: 39.1, Fiber: 12 g, Protein: 12.3 g.

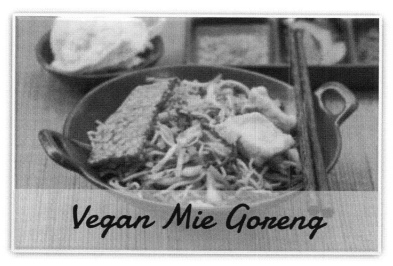

Vegan Mie Goreng

Serves 6 | Prep 15 min | Cook: 0 min | Ready in: 15 min

INGREDIENTS

1 cup chopped napa cabbage
1 cup Spinach
½ c. bean sprouts
1 cup sliced scallions
8 large cloves of garlic, minced
2 tablespoons sesame oil
1/4 cup soy sauce
3 tablespoons olive oil
1 tsp red pepper flakes
1 lb vegan noodles
4 oz tofu
4 oz tempeh
Salt and Pepper
Sweet Chili sauce

DIRECTIONS

1. Boil the noodles according to the package instructions.
2. Heat the oil in a large skillet. Add the scallions and saute until translucent (about 3 minutes). Add the garlic, cabbage, spinach and bean sprouts. Satue until the vegetables just start to get tender and spinach is wilted (about 2 minutes). Remove the vegetables from the pan and place on a plate.
3. Heat another tbsp. of oil in the skillet and once it's nice and hot, add the tofu and tempeh searing on all sides.
4. Add the vegetables back in and add all remaining ingredient. Stir until well combined and heated through.

PREPPING

Portion the noodles into 4 meal prep dishes, and store in the fridge for up to 4 days. Heat in the microwave before eating.

NUTRITION PER SERVING:

Calories: 401, Fat: 26.2 g Carbs: 31.1, Fiber: 3.7 g, Protein: 14.1 g.

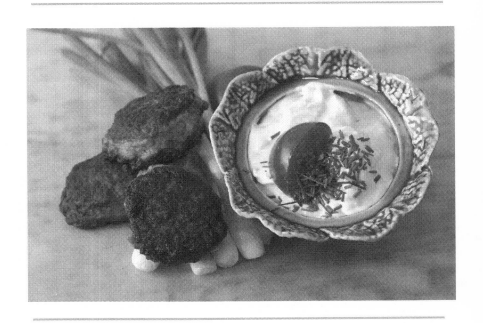

Freezer Meals

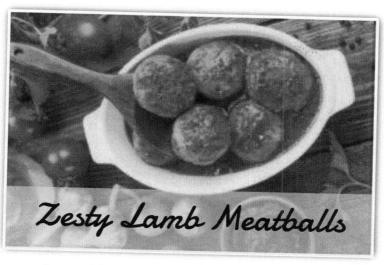

Zesty Lamb Meatballs

Serves 4 | Prep 15 min | Cook: 20 min | Ready in: 35 min

INGREDIENTS

1 lb. of ground lamb
1 large egg
1 tsp of fennel seed
1 tsp of salt
2 tsp of crushed garlic
1 tsp of pepper
1 tsp of paprika
2 tbsp. of coconut oil
1 onion, diced small

DIRECTIONS

1. In a large bowl combine all the ingredients except the additional ones.
2. Shape into a dozen meatballs then put aside.
3. Heat the coconut oil and onion in a pan for eight to ten minutes.
4. Add the garlic and heat for another couple of minutes.
5. Add the meatballs and cook until there is no pink showing on any side. They should be firm to the touch.

Prepping

Take off the heat, cool quickly and portion off. Put in the freezer until ready for a meal. The food will keep for six months in the freezer. You can heat up by baking at 350, or by microwaving them in a glass dish with a little bit of water.

Nutrition Per Serving:

Calories: 303, Fat: 16.5 g Carbs: 3.6, Fiber: 1.1 g, Protein: 33.9 g.

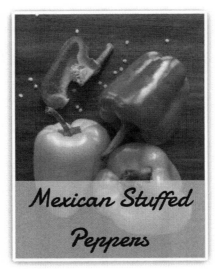

Mexican Stuffed Peppers

Serves 6 | Prep 15 min | Cook: 30 min | Ready in: 45 min

INGREDIENTS

1-1/2 lb. lean ground turkey
1 large onion, chopped small
2 garlic cloves, minced
6 small green bell peppers, tops cut off and cleaned out (seeds and pulp removed)
1 (10 oz) can diced tomatoes w/green chilies
1/4 c. fresh cilantro, chopped
1 (1.25 oz.) packet of taco seasoning
1/2 tsp. cumin
1/2 tsp. salt
1/4 tsp. fresh ground pepper
2 c. medium salsa
1c. shredded mozzarella cheese

DIRECTIONS

1. Mix the ground turkey, onion, garlic, canned diced tomatoes, cilantro, taco seasoning, cumin, salt and pepper. Mix until completely combined.
2. Spoon the meat mixture into the topless green peppers (make sure to portion evenly).

PREPPING

Wrap each pepper in plastic, then Freeze the peppers in a large freezer bag. When you're ready to eat them, transfer the peppers into a baking dish. Bake at 350 in the oven until they're fully cooked. Top with salsa and mozzarella. And put them back in the oven until the cheese melts.

Nutrition Per Serving:

Calories: 219, Fat: 7.6 g Carbs: 20.8, Fiber: 4.2 g, Protein: 20.4 g.

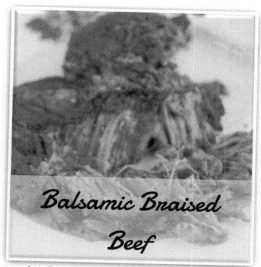

Balsamic Braised Beef

Serves **6** | Prep **10 min** | Cook: **8 HRS** | Ready in: **8 HRS**

INGREDIENTS

3 pound boneless roast beef (chuck or round roast)
Kosher salt and pepper
1/4 cup balsamic vinegar
1 cup beef stock
2 tablespoons soy sauce
1 tablespoon honey
4 cloves garlic, minced, fine
½ teaspoon red pepper flakes (increase if you want more heat)

DIRECTIONS

1. Simply combine all ingredients in a large freezer bag and squish the liquid around coating the beef.
2. Freeze in the bag

PREPPING

The night before you're ready to enjoy this meal, remove the bag from the freezer and put it in the fridge to defrost. The next morning, pour the contents of the bag into the slow cooker and cook on low for 8 hours. (great for a busy day at work). When the meat is done cooking, take 2 forks and shred the beef.

Nutrition Per Serving:

Calories: **337**, Fat: **13.3 g** Carbs: **3.4**, Fiber: **0.1 g**, Protein: **47.6 g**.

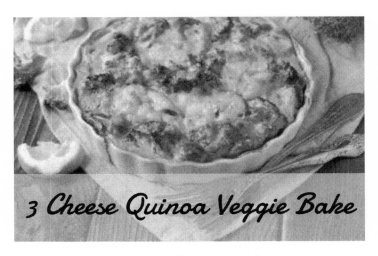

3 Cheese Quinoa Veggie Bake

Serves 5 | Prep 20 min | Cook: 30 min | Ready in: 50 min

INGREDIENTS

2 tablespoons olive oil
1 cup finely chopped broccoli
1 cup finely chopped cauliflower
1 cup Zucchini, cut into half moons
2 cup fresh spinach
4 garlic cloves, minced
1 yellow onion
1/2 teaspoon ground thyme
1/2 tsp rosemary, dried
1/2 teaspoon Italian seasoning
½ tsp. kosher salt
¼ tsp. fresh ground black pepper
2 cups cooked quinoa
1 cup Greek yogurt
1 1/2 cups chicken broth
1/2 cup grated parmesan
2/3 cup shredded cheddar cheese
2/3 cup mozzarella cheese

Nutrition Per Serving:

Calories: 353, Fat: 19.2 g Carbs: 25, Fiber: 4 g, Protein: 22.5 g.

DIRECTIONS

1. Heat oil in a large skillet, then add in the zucchini, cauliflower, broccoli, and spinach and onion and garlic. Stir until vegetables start to get tender and spinach is wilted (about 5 minutes). Stir and make sure garlic doesn't stick to the bottom and scorch. Add the thyme, rosemary, Italian seasoning, salt and pepper and stir and remove from heat. Stir in the quinoa
2. In a bowl, whisk together the greek yogurt, chicken broth and parmesan until well combined. Stir in 1/3 cup of cheddar cheese and 1/3 cup of mozzarella.
3. Combine the yogurt mixture and the quinoa veggie mixture and spread in a greased baking dish.
4. Top with the remaining 1/3 cup of cheddar cheese and 1/3 cup of mozzarella.

Prepping

1. Carefully wrap the baking dish with plastic, and then again with foil so it is completely sealed and air tight. Place in the freezer.
2. The night before you want to eat this dish, thaw in the fridge overnight. The next day bake at 375 degrees F, for about 30 minutes or until the top is golden and slightly crispy and the sides are bubbly.

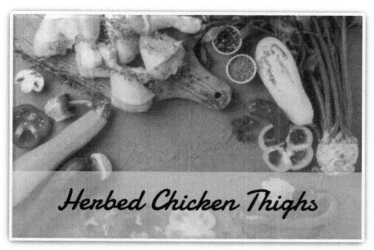

Herbed Chicken Thighs

Serves 4 | Prep 10 min | Cook 30 min | Ready in: 40 min

INGREDIENTS

4 boneless chicken thighs, with the skin on
2 zucchinis
½ cup of sliced carrots
2 tbsp. of olive oil
2 tbsp. of balsamic vinegar
(1) 1-inch cube of ginger, minced
1 tsp Italian Seasoning
Salt and Pepper to taste

DIRECTIONS

1. Season chicken with salt pepper and Italian seasoning.
2. Arrange the thighs on a greased baking tray.
3. Slice all the vegetables and arrange them around the chicken.
4. Mix the oil, vinegar and ginger, and spread over the food.
5. Bake for thirty minutes at 350 degrees F.

PREPPING

1. Cool quickly, divide up into portions. Freeze.
2. Defrost and reheat in the microwave until piping hot. Serve with mashed potatoes or a garden salad
3. This meal will keep for three to six months in the freezer.

NUTRITION PER SERVING:

Calories: 187, Fat: 11.2 g Carbs: 4.7, Fiber: 1.4 g, Protein: 17.1 g.

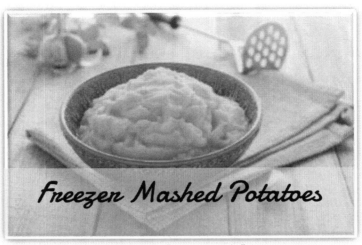

Freezer Mashed Potatoes

Serves 6 | Prep 5 min | Cook: 15 min | Ready in: 20 min

INGREDIENTS

3 pounds red skin potatoes, peeled and diced
3 tablespoons butter
4 ounces sour cream
1/2 Cup Half and Half
Kosher Salt
Black Pepper

DIRECTIONS

1. Place the diced potatoes in a pot and cover with water. Bring to a boil and continue to boil until the potatoes are fork tender (about 15 minutes).
2. Add all remaining ingredients and use a potato masher to mash the potatoes and completely mix all the ingredients. Continue adding cream until you've reached your desired consistency.

Prepping

1. Once the potatoes have cooled to room temperature, scoop them into large freezer bags and freeze.
2. Before eating, you can either thaw in the fridge or in the microwave. Add a bit of milk if needed.

Nutrition Per Serving:

Calories: 244, Fat: 6.6 g Carbs: 40.7, Fiber: 3.6 g, Protein: 5.8 g.

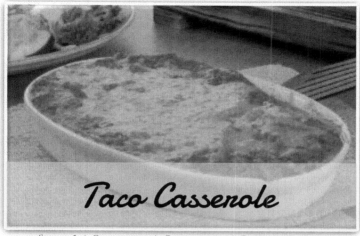

Taco Casserole

Serves 6 | Prep 15 min | Cook: 45 min | Ready in: 60 min

INGREDIENTS

1 pound of ground turkey
1 onion chopped
1 cup of corn
1 (14 oz) cans of black beans, drained but not rinsed.
2 cans of diced tomatoes with green chilis
¼ c. taco seasoning
2 c. brown rice, cooked
1 cup salsa
2/3 cup of shredded Mexican Cheese

DIRECTIONS

1. In a skillet over medium heat, brown the ground turkey. Add the onions and saute until translucent and tender. Add in the taco seasoning and ¼ cup of water. Simmer until water has cooked off (about 7 minutes)
2. Stir in the corn, canned tomatoes, black beans
3. Grease a baking dish, and spread the rice in the bottom, then top with the taco meat mixture, then top with the salsa and sprinkle the cheese on top

PREPPING

1. Wrap tightly with plastic wrap and then wrap again with foil completely all around the pan. Freeze
2. When you want to eat the dish, thaw overnight in the fridge. Before eating, bake at 350 degrees for about 45 minutes (until top is golden and sides are bubbly).

Nutrition Per Serving:

Calories: 266, Fat: 8.3 g Carbs: 27.2, Fiber: 3.9 g, Protein: 24.2 g.

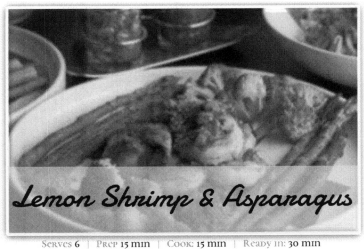

Lemon Shrimp & Asparagus

Serves 6 | Prep 15 min | Cook: 15 min | Ready in: 30 min

INGREDIENTS

12 asparagus stalks, cut into two-inch sections
2 tablespoons of butter
1 ½ lbs. of shrimp
1 tsp of lemon pepper
1 tsp. lemon zest
2 cloves of crushed garlic
½ tsp of salt
Lemon wedges (for serving)

DIRECTIONS

1. In a large bowl, place the shrimp and add half of the butter. Sprinkle on the lemon pepper, lemon zest, add the garlic and toss with a little salt.
2. Add the shrimps to the tray, pushing the asparagus to one end.
3. Cook for another seven or eight minutes.

Prepping

1. Cool and freeze.
2. When ready to serve, heat the shrimp in the sauce over the stove. Serve over cauliflower rice or tofu noodles
3. Make the Asparagus the day of: Preheat the oven to 400 degrees. Spread the asparagus in a layer on a tray and drizzle with half of the melted butter. Add a dash of salt and pepper and toss the asparagus.
4. Bake for four minutes.
5. I like to serve this dish with tofu noodles. They taste like regular noodles but have almost no calories. Look for shirataki noodles in the supermarket.
6. This meal will keep for three to six months in the freezer.

Nutrition Per Serving:

Calories: 266, Fat: 8.3 g Carbs: 27.2, Fiber: 3.9 g, Protein: 24.2 g.

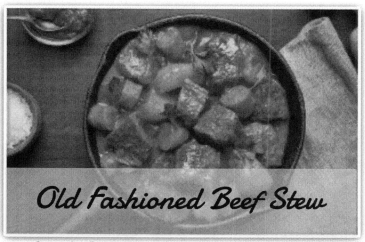

Old Fashioned Beef Stew

Serves 6 | Prep 20 min | Cook: 30 min | Ready in: 60 min

INGREDIENTS

1 lb. of beef for stewing, chopped into bite sized pieces
2 cups of beef broth
4 cloves of crushed garlic
1 diced onion
1 chopped up yellow pepper
2 cups of chunky carrots
2 cups of chunky radish
A pinch of salt and pepper
½ tsp. Corn starch (to thicken if necessary)
1 tbsp. of butter
1 tbsp. of coconut oil

DIRECTIONS

1. Heat a large pan and add the coconut oil. Brown the beef on all sides, then move aside.
2. Add the onions and garlic to the pan, plus the butter, and cook for two to three minutes. Scrape the bottom of the pan to keep those flavoursome pieces.
3. Add the broth and cornstarch
4. When the mixture comes to the boil, add the beef back in. Simmer for thirty minutes
5. Add the vegetables and cook for another thirty minutes. Add water if the stew begins to dry out.

Prepping

1. Cool and freeze. You can either freeze in a freezer bag or in a large plastic container. Simply reheat on the Stove top when you want to eat it.
2. This will keep for six months in the freezer.

Nutrition Per Serving:

Calories: 330, Fat: 14.1 g Carbs: 11.2, Fiber: 2.9 g, Protein: 38.1 g.

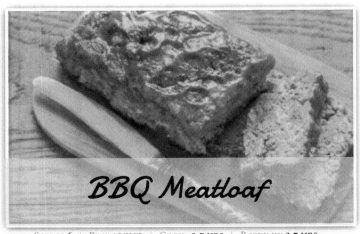

BBQ Meatloaf

Serves 6 | Prep 15 min | Cook: 3-7 HRS | Ready in: 3-7 HRS

INGREDIENTS

1 1/2 pounds lean ground beef
2 eggs
1/2 c. milk
1/4 c. water
1 medium yellow onion chopped
1/2 c. grated parmesan cheese
(the powdery dry kind that
comes in a can)
1 teaspoon salt
1/4 tsp ground black pepper
1 c. sliced mushrooms
2 tbsp. ketchup
1 tbsp brown sugar
2 tbsp. Dijon mustard
1/2 teaspoon Worcestershire
sauce
1c. prepared BBQ Sauce

DIRECTIONS

1. Combine all ingredients in a large mixing bowl and stir together. Use your hands to combine the ingredients and make sure everything is evenly incorporated
2. Form a loaf with the meat mixture and place in the slow cooker. Brush the top with ½ c. of the bbq sauce.

PREPPING

1. Place the meatloaf in a large freezer bag and freeze.

2. The day before you want to eat this dish, remove from the freezer and thaw in the fridge overnight.

3. Place the meatloaf in the slow cooker and Cook on low for 6-7 hours of high for 3-4.

4. 15 minutes before serving, brush on the rest of the BBQ sauce. Serve with extra BBQ if desired.

Nutrition Per Serving:

Calories: **289**, Fat: **10.7 g** Carbs: **17.8**, Fiber: **0.6 g**, Protein: **29.5 g**.

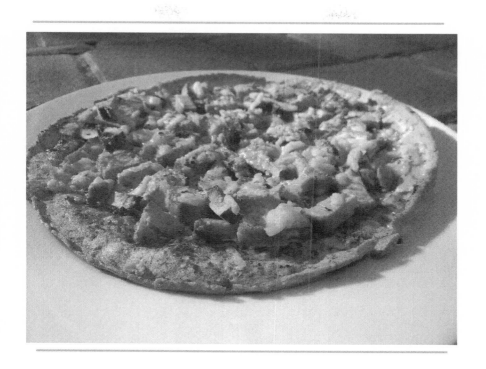

Paleo Style

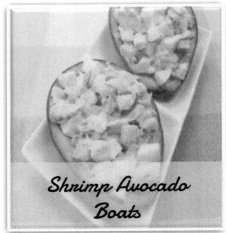

Shrimp Avocado Boats

INGREDIENTS

2 avocados
Lime juice
1 pound shrimp
2 cloves garlic, minced
1/8 red onion
1/2 c. chopped cucumber (optional)
1/2 tsp. fresh dill, chopped.
1/4 c. Paleo mayonnaise (homemade if you cannot find in grocery store)

DIRECTIONS

1. Cut the shrimp roughly into small pieces. Sear the shrimp with the minced garlic in your cast iron skillet until golden brown. Cut the avocado in half and take out the seed. Chop up the red onion to small bits and mix them into the shrimp. Make sure that they are sautéed for a few minutes. Remove from heat and add mayo, cucumber, dill and lime juice and mix with the shrimp.
2. When the avocado is cut, the outside part of it will begin to oxidize. To delay this from happening, squirt more lime juice onto the avocado itself.
3. Next place the shrimp into the avocado where the seed used to be, and serve.

PREPPING

making the shrimp mixture ahead—add extra lemon or lime juice to keep it fresh. Store it in glass for up to 3 days. Cut the avocado and stuff it right before eating.

NUTRITION PER SERVING:

Calories: 241, Fat: 11.1 g Carbs: 8.5, Fiber: 3.1 g, Protein: 27 g.

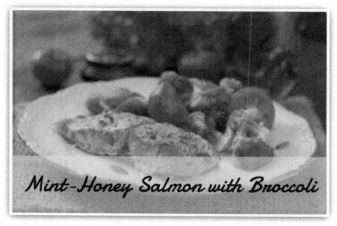

Mint-Honey Salmon with Broccoli

Serves 4 | Prep 15 min | Cook: 20 min | Ready in: 35 min

INGREDIENTS

2 pounds salmon filet
2 cloves garlic
¼ teaspoon pepper
2 teaspoons fresh mint leaves
2 lemons
2 tbsp. Olive oil
2 crowns broccoli
3 tablespoons honey

DIRECTIONS

1. Mince garlic and chop broccoli into pieces. In a cast iron skillet, pour some olive oil and add chopped broccoli and some of the garlic. Sauté until the broccoli is bright green. Add a dash of lemon or salt to taste.

2. Season salmon with salt, pepper, garlic, and lemon juice. Pour olive oil onto another cast iron skillet and add the salmon. Continue seasoning the salmon with salt and lemon juice while it is cooking. Turn it over and lightly season the other side.

3. In a separate bowl, mince the rest of the garlic, and add lemon juice and honey. Baste this over the salmon while it is cooking. Serve warm with the broccoli and refrigerate separately

PREPPING

This whole dish is good reheated for 2-3 days. Store in glass and I recommend heating the salmon in the oven or stove top. If you want to try the microwave, add a few tsp of water to the dish to keep it from drying out.

Nutrition Per Serving:

Calories: 414, Fat: 19.8 g Carbs: 18.2, Fiber: 1.9 g, Protein: 41.3 g.

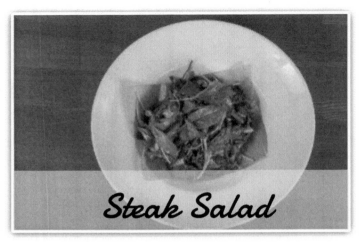

Steak Salad

Serves **6** | Prep **15 min** | Cook: **5 min** | Ready in: **20 min**

INGREDIENTS

½ teaspoon sea salt
½ teaspoon pepper
¼ teaspoon garlic powder
24 ounces steak
¼ cup olive oil
Lemon juice
1 teaspoon Dijon mustard
4 cups arugula
½ cup red onion
1 red bell pepper sliced thin
½ avocado

DIRECTIONS

1. Chop the onion and dice the avocado. Cut the steak into four equal-sized pieces. Combine the spices together into a mixture and rub them over the steak until it absorbs the spices.
2. In your cast iron skillet, add the seasoned steak. Use little olive oil. This is done to sear and blacken the steak. Once the steak is medium-rare (about 5 minutes into the cooking), place it on a cutting board and cut into thin slices. OR just cook longer to your desired level of "doneness."
3. Then combine some olive oil, mustard, and lemon juice in a large bowl. Add the blackened steak, arugula, avocado and chopped onion to the salad. Serve hot or cold.

Prepping

Cook the steak and mix all of the dry ingredients of the salad. Add the avocado and dressing and place the sliced cooked steak on top of the salad just before eating. Alternatively, to make sure you have a fresh hot steak every night you eat the salad, you can prepare everything and mix together the dressing, then cook the steak the night of (only takes 5 minutes). While the steak is searing, dress the salad, and slice and add the avocado. Dinner will be ready in 5 minutes.

Nutrition Per Serving:

Calories: **340**, Fat: **17.5 g** Carbs: **3.1**, Fiber: **1.6 g**, Protein: **41.8 g**.

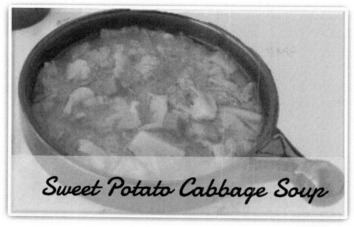

Sweet Potato Cabbage Soup

Serves 6 | Prep 15 min | Cook: 5 min | Ready in: 20 min

INGREDIENTS

2 tsp. ghee (or olive oil)
1 small onion
1 pound ground beef
6 shiitake mushrooms
2 garlic cloves
6 cups bone broth
1 crown cabbage
2 large carrots
1 sweet potato
Black pepper
Sea salt

PREPPING

store in glass in the fridge for up to 4 days. Simply heat and eat. You can easily just heat it in a microwave safe dish at work. How easy is that? Great for cold weather when you're craving comfort food.

DIRECTIONS

1. Dice the onion, mince the garlic, and peel and cut the carrots. Cut the sweet potato into inch long cubes. Cut the cabbage into thin squares and dice the mushrooms. Make sure to stem the mushrooms before you chop them up.
2. In a large pot, heat up the ghee over medium heat. Then throw in the onions and stir until they are tender. Then add the ground beef and mushrooms and continue to sauté for another 6 minutes. Until the beef is cooked and there is no pink left. Next, add the garlic and stir until fragrant (about 2 minutes).
3. Add the broth to the pot.
4. Turn up the heat stirring until the broth is boiling. Once bubbles are forming, add the sweet potato, cabbage, and carrots. Bring heat down to a simmer and partially cover the pot with a lid for another 15-30 minutes or until the beef is completely cooked and the vegetables are completely soft and tender. Season with salt and pepper.

NUTRITION PER SERVING:

Calories: 256, Fat: 6.6 g Carbs: 24.6, Fiber: 6 g, Protein: 26.3 g.

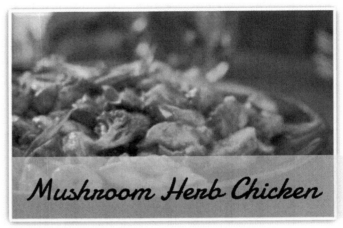

Mushroom Herb Chicken

Serves 4 | Prep 10 min | Cook: 20 min | Ready in: 30 min

INGREDIENTS

4 chicken breast halves sliced into 1 inch cubes
1/4 teaspoon salt and pepper
Olive oil
Lemon juice
3 Shallots (can also use scallions)
1 cup broccoli
1 cup thin slices bell pepper (red or orange or yellow)
1 package mushrooms
1/3 cup red wine vinegar
½ Tsp. dried Italian seasoning
½ tbsp. fresh Thyme

Prepping

Keeps well in glass in the Refrigerator for up to 5 days.

DIRECTIONS

1. Season chicken with salt and pepper while drizzling with olive oil. Heat a cast iron skillet to medium high and add the seasoned chicken. Cook until light brown on both sides. Add lemon juice as needed.
2. While the chicken is cooking, cut the shallots and mix with mushrooms and broccoli and the peppers and the Italian seasoning and the thyme.
3. Once chicken is done cooking, add some more olive oil to the skillet and sauté the mushrooms, broccoli, and shallots. Then add in the chicken to mix them all together until the broccoli and mushrooms are well cooked.

Nutrition Per Serving:

Calories: 234, Fat: 10.3 g Carbs: 5.2, Fiber: 1.4 g, Protein: 29.3 g.

Healthy Desserts

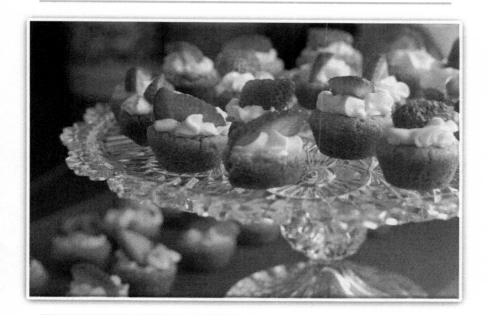

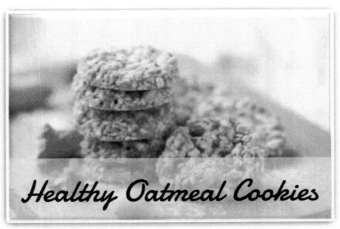

Healthy Oatmeal Cookies

Serves **8** | Prep **25** min | Cook: **20** min | Ready in: **45** min

INGREDIENTS

1/2 c. whole-wheat flour
1/4 c. all-purpose flour
1/2 c. granulated sugar
1/2 tsp. ground cinnamon
1 pinch Kosher salt
1 c. quick-cooking oats
1 c. unsweetened shredded coconut
1/2 c. walnuts
1/4 c. golden raisins
1/4 c. dried cranberries
1/2 c. unsalted butter
3 tbsp. Honey
1/2 tsp. baking soda
3 tbsp. boiling water

Nutrition Per Serving:

Calories: **343**, Fat: **19.4** g Carbs: **40.7**, Fiber: **2.8** g, Protein: **5** g.

Note: Servings size is 2 cookies because they're so good you won't be able to just eat one.

DIRECTIONS

1. Sift together flour sugar cinnamon and salt in a large bowl. Stir in the coconut, walnuts, raisins cranberries and oats.
2. In a saucepan, melt the butter, stir in the honey, meanwhile, in a mug, microwave the 3tbps of water until boiling, stir in the baking soda to the hot water, then add this to the honey mixture.
3. Add the wet ingredients to the dry mixing until just combined (do not overmix).
4. Roll the dough into balls and flatten them slightly.
5. Bake at 350 for 17-20 minutes or until the edges are golden and the center is cooked.

Prepping

1. There are a few ways you can do this: make the dough and store it in an air tight container in the fridge for up to 5 days and make the cookies in batches or at a later time, OR make the cookies and just store them
2. These cookies freeze really well. All you have to do is pull a few out of the freezer and let them come to room temperature (it only takes a few minutes). Or for a warm treat, just sprinkle a few drops of water on them and microwave them for 10-20 seconds and they will be soft and warm.

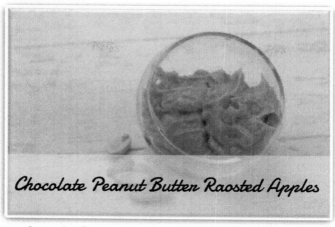

Chocolate Peanut Butter Raosted Apples

Serves **6** | Prep **5 min** | Cook: **15 min** | Ready in: **20 min**

INGREDIENTS

3 apples, cored and halved
1tbps butter, melted
1 cup peanut butter
1/2 cup semisweet chocolate chips

DIRECTIONS

1. Place the apples in a baking dish and brush them with butter.
2. Bake at 375 for 15 minutes
3. Portion out the peanut butter evenly into each apple half

Prepping

at this point, store the peanut butter apples in the fridge for up to 2 days on a glass plate covered with foil or plastic. When you're ready to eat, bake them at 375 for 15 more minutes. Meanwhile, melt the chocolate in the microwave. Once the apples are done, drizzle with melted chocolate and enjoy.

Nutrition Per Serving:

Calories: **438**, Fat: **31 g** Carbs: **35.9**, Fiber: **6.3 g**, Protein: **11.1 g**.

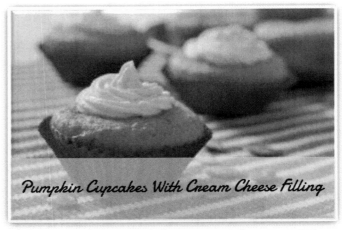

Pumpkin Cupcakes With Cream Cheese Filling

Serves 20 | Prep 25 min | Cook: 25 min | Ready in: 50 min

INGREDIENTS

1 cup pumpkin puree
6 eggs
2 tbsp sour cream
2 tbsp butter
1 tbsp pumpkin pie spice
½ cup flour
½ cup coconut oil
1 ½ tsp baking powder
1 ½ tsp vanilla
½ tsp salt
1/4 c. honey

For Filling:
½ tsp vanilla
1 tbsp heavy whipped cream
3 oz cream cheese
2 tbsp. sugar

Nutrition Per Serving:

Calories: 131, Fat: 10 g Carbs: 8.8,
Fiber: 0.5 g, Protein: 2.5 g.

DIRECTIONS

1. Preheat oven to 350 degrees F.
2. Place a pan over medium-low heat and melt the butter and coconut oil.
3. Crack the eggs in a mixing bowl and add the pumpkin puree, vanilla, sour cream and pumpkin spice and honey. Whisk the mixture well.
4. Pour the melted butter and coconut oil over the mixture.
5. Take a separate mixing bowl and mix the coconut flour, baking powder, and salt.
6. Pour the flour mixture into the first mixing bowl. Mix thoroughly.
7. Make the filling by pouring its ingredients into a blender. Mix well.
8. Grease muffin tins, line them with parchment paper, and then fill them with the batter.
9. Use a spoon to scoop the filling over the top of the batter of each muffin tin. Leave about half of the filling for later.
10. Use a toothpick to swirl the filling into the batter.
11. Place in the oven for 25 minutes.

Prepping

1. You can easily freeze these, or else store them in the fridge for up to 5 days.
2. Before serving, top off with the remaining cream filling.

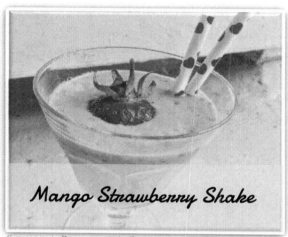

Mango Strawberry Shake

Serves 4 | Prep 5 min | Cook: 0 min | Ready in: 5 min

INGREDIENTS

1 banana
1 cup frozen strawberries
1 cup frozen mango
1 cup Greek yogurt
1/2 cup almond milk (or soy or cow)
1/4 tsp. ground cinnamon (optional)

DIRECTIONS

1. Combine all ingredients in blender and pulse until smooth and completely blended.

Prepping

you can make this smoothie ahead and store in a glass jar in the fridge for up to 3 days.

Nutrition Per Serving:

Calories: 171, Fat: 8.4 g Carbs: 20, Fiber: 2.9 g, Protein: 6.4 g.

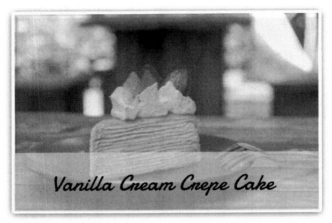

Vanilla Cream Crepe Cake

Serves **6** | Prep **10 min** | Cook: **20 min** | Ready in: **30 min**

INGREDIENTS

For the Crepes:
2 large eggs
¼ cup flour
2 tbsp butter
2 oz cream cheese
1 tsp unsweetened soy milk
2 tbsp. sugar

For The Topping And Filling;
6 large strawberries
½ tsp vanilla extract
4 oz heavy cream
½ c. powdered sugar

PREPPING

Store the cake in the fridge, covered for up to 4 days. Slice and serve chilled.

Nutrition Per Serving:

Calories: **236**, Fat: **15.9 g** Carbs: **20.3**, Fiber: **0.5 g**, Protein: **3.9 g**.

DIRECTIONS

1. The first step is to make the batter for the crepes. Break the eggs into a food processor and then add the cream cheese and almond flour. Mix the ingredients well. Pour in the soy milk and process the ingredients until you get a smooth consistency. Add more soy milk if necessary, to thin the mixture.
2. Place a frying pan over medium heat. Melt some of the butter in the pan and grease the surface evenly. When the butter becomes hot, pour two tablespoons of the batter into the pan and swirl it to ensure a thin layer.
3. When the edges of the crepe turn brown, use a spatula to flip it over to the other side. Cook until the crepe turns slightly brown and then remove it from the pan.
4. Use the remaining batter to make the rest of the crepes. There should be enough to make five more. Allow all the crepes to cool.
5. As the crepes cool, prepare the filling. Pour the heavy cream and vanilla extract and sugar into the bowl of an electric mixter and whip on high until the cream forms soft peaks.
6. Arrange the crepes in a neat stack and then use a sharp knife to cut the stack in half.
7. Take one crepe (or rather half-crepe) and place it on a serving plate. Spread some of the cream and vanilla filling over the top of the crepe, making sure that it is a thin layer. Take another crepe, stack it on top of the first one, and spread another thin layer of filling. Repeat the process until you have used all the crepes.
8. When you are done, put the crepes in the fridge for about an hour.
9. Meanwhile, slice the strawberries into halves.
10. After one hour, remove the crepes and top off with some whipped cream and the halved strawberries.

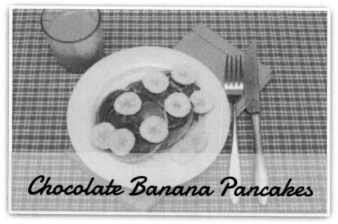

Chocolate Banana Pancakes

Serves 4 | Prep 10 min | Cook: 20 min | Ready in: 30 min

INGREDIENTS

3 large and ripe bananas
4 eggs
Olive oil spray
¼ teaspoon baking powder
¼ c. powdered sugar
½ Semisweet chocolate chips

DIRECTIONS

1. Crack the four eggs and mix them together in a bowl. Once they are mixed, add the baking powder to the mixture. In a separate bowl, lightly mash the three large and ripe bananas until they are mush. Pour the egg batter into the mashed bananas slowly. Continue to stir until the two mixtures are combined and the batter thickens up a bit. Then stir in the powdered sugar

2. In your cast iron skillet, lightly spray some olive oil to cover the skillet and its edges. Add dollops of batter to the cast iron skillet. Make sure to space them out well enough so that they do not touch. If your skillet is too small, you may have to make one or two pancakes at a time. Once the bottom is light brown, flip the pancake to heat the other side.

3. In a separate bowl, lightly microwave the chocolate chips until they are completely melted. Depending on the thickness of the chocolate, you can spread it on top of the pancakes or just drizzle it if it is thin enough.

Prepping

1. You can freeze these pancakes and simply microwave them and drizzle with chocolate for a midnight snack or a light dessert.
2. Refrigerate pancakes for up to five days, but make sure to only melt the chocolate and drizzle the pancakes right before you are about to eat.

Nutrition Per Serving:

Calories: **312**, Fat: **12.8 g** Carbs: **46.2**, Fiber: **3.8 g**, Protein: **6.5 g**.

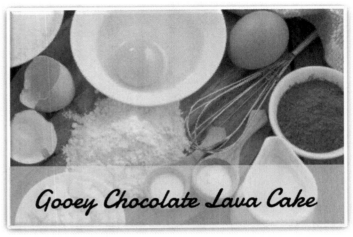

Gooey Chocolate Lava Cake

Serves **8** | Prep **10** min | Cook: **20** min | Ready in: **30** min

INGREDIENTS

1/3 c. cocoa powder (unsweetened)

1/2 c. all purpose flour (use GF if preferred)

1 1/2 cup sugar substitute (use a Stevia-Erythritol blend)

1 tsp. baking powder

1/2 tsp. salt

1/2 c. (1 stick) salted butter melted

3 eggs

3 egg yolks

1 tsp. vanilla extract

1/2 c. sugar-free chocolate chips

2 c. hot water

Cooking Spray

Frozen Sugar-free whipped topping, thawed

DIRECTIONS

1. Sift together the sweetener, flour, cocoa, salt, baking powder in a medium bowl. Add the melted butter and stir, then add the eggs, egg yolks and vanilla extract. Stir until combined (do not beat or overmix).
2. Lightly grease the crockpot with a no-cal cooking spray (make sure it is not flavored). Then pour in the chocolate batter. Scatter the chocolate chips evenly over the batter, then pour in the two cups of hot water
3. Cook on low for 3 hrs.

PREPPING

1. Store in the fridge for up to 4 days. Scoop out a helping and microwave it and enjoy.
2. Top with thawed whipped topping if desired.

Nutrition Per Serving:

Calories: **256**, Fat: **19.6 g** Carbs: **18**, Fiber: **1.3 g**, Protein: **5.7 g**.

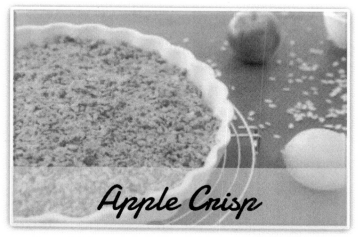

Apple Crisp

Serves **8** | Prep **10 min** | Cook: **20 min** | Ready in: **30 min**

INGREDIENTS

1/2 cup firmly packed brown sugar
1/2 cup honey
1 cup almond flour
1/2 cup flour
1 cup old fashioned oats
1/4 tsp cinnamon
1/8 tsp nutmeg opt.
4 tbsp butter melted
½ banana mashed.
2 1/2 cups sliced apples

DIRECTIONS

1. Melt the butter, and meanwhile in a large bowl, whisk together the almond flour, all purpose flour, oats, cinnamon, nutmeg, and brown sugar.
2. In a separate small bowl, mix together the melted butter, mashed banana and honey, until smooth and liquidy and completely combined. Then add to the flour mixture and mix until completely incorporated and crumbly.
3. Spread apple slices out in a greased baking dish and sprinlkle on the oat mixture mixing in slightly until apples are completely covered.
4. Bake at 350 degrees F, until the top is golden brown and the apples are completely tender.

Prepping

This dessert freezes great! You can simply reheat covered with foil in the oven. Top with a dollop of fat free whipped topping.

Nutrition Per Serving:

Calories: **256**, Fat: **19.6 g** Carbs: **18**, Fiber: **1.3 g**, Protein: **5.7 g**.

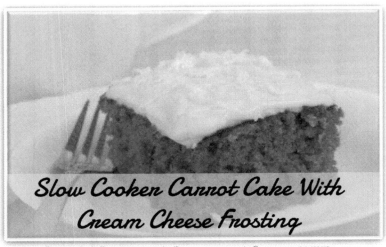

Slow Cooker Carrot Cake With Cream Cheese Frosting

Serves **8** | Prep **10 min** | Cook: **20 min** | Ready in: **30 min**

INGREDIENTS

3/4 c. sugar substitute (use a Stevia-Erythritol blend)
1/2 c. vanilla protein powder
1-1/2 c. flour
1/4 tsp. salt
2 tsp. baking powder
1-1/2 tsp. ground cinnamon
1/4 tsp. ground nutmeg
1-1/2 c. grated carrots
3/4 c. unsweetened applesauce
4 eggs
3 tbsp. vegetable oil
1 tsp. vanilla extract
1/4 c. chopped pecans (optional)

Cream Cheese Frosting:
1 (8oz.) package Neufchâtel (cream) cheese
3 tbsp. butter
1/3 c. powdered sugar
1 tsp. vanilla extract

DIRECTIONS

1. Sift together sweetener, protein powder, almond flour salt, baking powder, cinnamon, and nutmeg. In a separate bowl, whisk together carrots, applesauce, eggs, oil and vanilla extract. Combine the wet and dry ingredients and stir until just mixed. Do not overbeat.
2. Grease the crockpot and either dust with flour or line with waxed paper.
3. Pour in the carrot cake batter, and spread evenly. Cook on low for 3 hours (test with a toothpick).
4. While the cake is cooking, beat the Neufchâtel cheese and butter together (it really helps if the butter and cream cheese are at room temperature and soft) in a standing mixer or in a medium bowl with a hand mixer. Beat until the mixture is light and fluffy. Slowly add in the sweetener while continuing to beat the mixture. Add in the vanilla and continue to beat until there are no lumps and the frosting is completely smooth. If you need to thin it out, use a few teaspoons of milk until at the desired consistency.
5. When the cake is mostly cooled, frost with the cream cheese frosting. Scatter the chopped pecans over the frosting and serve.

Prepping

This dessert freezes great! You can simply reheat covered with foil in the oven. Top with a dollop of fat free whipped topping.

Nutrition Per Serving:

Calories: **282**, Fat: **17.2 g** Carbs: **18.6**, Fiber: **1.5 g**, Protein: **14.9 g**.

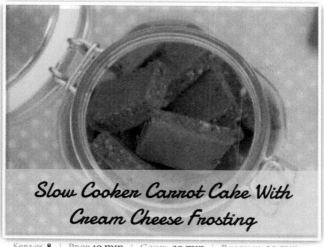

Slow Cooker Carrot Cake With Cream Cheese Frosting

Serves **8** | Prep **10 min** | Cook: **20 min** | Ready in: **30 min**

INGREDIENTS

3/4 cup sweet potato puree
1 tsp vanilla extract
1 cup natural peanut butter
1/4 cup flour
1/2 cup dark chocolate chips
2/3 cup granulated sugar
1/4 cup
1 1/2 tsp baking soda
1/8 tsp salt

DIRECTIONS

1. Microwave peanut butter until it's soft and liquidy and then stir in the sweet potato puree and vanilla.
2. In a separate bowl, mix together all the rest of the ingredients, then slowly mix the dry ingredients in the sweet potato mixture.
3. Pour the batter into a well-greased baking pan, and bake at 325 degrees F, for about 20 minutes.

PREPPING

Store these in an airtight container for up to 5 days, or freeze and pull them out as needed. You can simply let the brownies come to room temperature before eating, or microwave them for a warm treat.

Nutrition Per Serving:

Calories: **229,** Fat: **12.3g** Carbs: **25.1,** Fiber: **25.1g,** Protein: **7.9 g.**

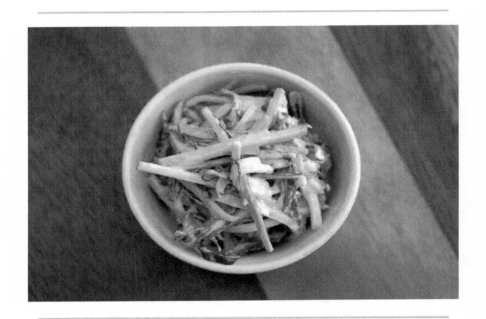

Side Dishes

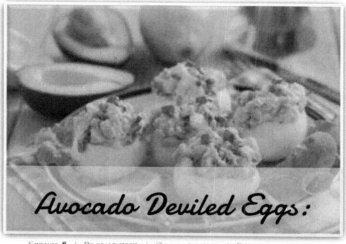

Avocado Deviled Eggs:

Serves **8** | Prep **10 min** | Cook: **20 min** | Ready in: **30 min**

INGREDIENTS

3 avocados
1 tomato
½ white onion;
½ cup chopped cilantro;
2 tbsp lemon juice
Salt and pepper to taste
6 eggs

DIRECTIONS

1. Finely dice the tomato, onion, and chop up the cilantro into small pieces. Cut the avocado into small pieces and mash it down with a fork. Stir in the other ingredients and sprinkle fresh lemon juice. This makes the guacamole.

2. Hard boil 6 eggs in water for 10 to 12 minutes. To hard boil and egg, put water in a pot until it begins to boil Make sure the pot is big enough to cover the eggs. Once the water's boiling, lower the eggs into the water. Then set the heater to a simmer. Once the timer for 10 to 12 minutes is up, remove the eggs. Take the crust off of the eggs and slice in half. Add guacamole to the eggs.

Prepping

Only cut up the eggs you want to immediately eat. Refrigerate the guacamole by wrapping it in a plastic wrap the physically touches the guacamole in order to stop it from turning brown. Alternatively, you can prepare the dish completely and consume within a few days and just spray lemon juice on the deviled eggs to keep the avocado from turning brown.

Nutrition Per Serving:

Calories: **211,** Fat: **17.8g** Carbs: **8.3,** Fiber: **6 g,** Protein: **7.4**

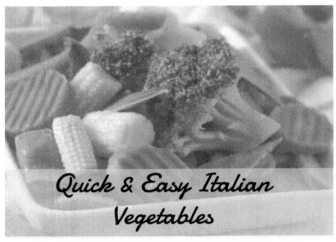

Quick & Easy Italian Vegetables

Serves **8** | Prep **10 min** | Cook: **20 min** | Ready in: **30 min**

INGREDIENTS

1 (10 oz) bag of California mix frozen vegetables
2 tbps. Grated parmesan
1 tbps. Butter
¼ tsp. Garlic Powder
½ tsp. Italian Seasoning
Salt and Pepper to Taste

DIRECTIONS

1. Steam the vegetables in the microwave according to the package directions (place them in a glass dish (covered with a few tbsp. of water).
2. Once the vegetables are steaming hot, pour off the water, and then add the rest of the ingredients. Mix until the butter is melted and all the vegetables are coated with the cheese and seasonings.

Prepping

while you can make this dish ahead and just store it in the fridge, it's so quick that you might as well just make it right before eating. Simply prep by keeping the ingredients on hand.

Nutrition Per Serving:

Calories: **88**, Fat: **4.9 g** Carbs: **7.2**, Fiber: **2.4 g**, Protein: **4.3**

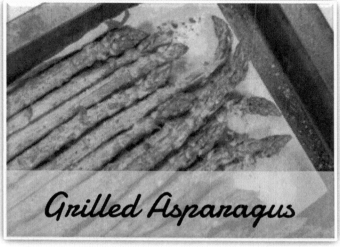

Grilled Asparagus

Serves **8** | Prep **10 min** | Cook: **20 min** | Ready in: **30 min**

INGREDIENTS

1 (10 oz) bag of California mix frozen vegetables
2 tbps. Grated parmesan
1 tbps. Butter
¼ tsp. Garlic Powder
½ tsp. Italian Seasoning
Salt and Pepper to Taste

DIRECTIONS

1. Steam the vegetables in the microwave according to the package directions (place them in a glass dish (covered with a few tbsp. of water).
2. Once the vegetables are steaming hot, pour off the water, and then add the rest of the ingredients. Mix until the butter is melted and all the vegetables are coated with the cheese and seasonings.

Prepping

while you can make this dish ahead and just store it in the fridge, it's so quick that you might as well just make it right before eating. Simply prep by keeping the ingredients on hand.

Nutrition Per Serving:

Calories: **88**, Fat: **4.9 g** Carbs: **7.2**, Fiber: **2.4 g**, Protein: **4.3**

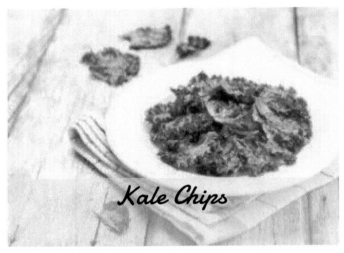

Kale Chips

Serves **8** | Prep **10 min** | Cook: **20 min** | Ready in: **30 min**

INGREDIENTS

1 (10 oz) bag of California mix frozen vegetables
2 tbps. Grated parmesan
1 tbps. Butter
¼ tsp. Garlic Powder
½ tsp. Italian Seasoning
Salt and Pepper to Taste

DIRECTIONS

1. Steam the vegetables in the microwave according to the package directions (place them in a glass dish (covered with a few tbsp. of water).
2. Once the vegetables are steaming hot, pour off the water, and then add the rest of the ingredients. Mix until the butter is melted and all the vegetables are coated with the cheese and seasonings.

Prepping

while you can make this dish ahead and just store it in the fridge, it's so quick that you might as well just make it right before eating. Simply prep by keeping the ingredients on hand.

Nutrition Per Serving:

Calories: **88**, Fat: **4.9 g** Carbs: **7.2**, Fiber: **2.4 g**, Protein: **4.3**

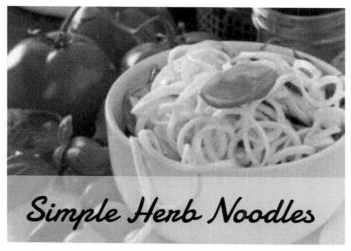

Simple Herb Noodles

Serves **8** | Prep **10 min** | Cook: **20 min** | Ready in: **30 min**

INGREDIENTS

2 zucchinis
1 tbsp. of olive oil
Salt and pepper
1 tbsp. butter
1 tbsp. Italian seasoning

DIRECTIONS

1. Spiralize the zucchinis and place them into a ziplock bag with tossed with the salt and Italian seasoning.

Prepping

Store the bag of zoodles in the fridge, and when you're ready to eat, heat the oil on the stove. Toss in the herbed zoodles. Stir until the vegetables are very tender (about 3-5 minutes). Top with 1 tbps butter and mix to coat.

Nutrition Per Serving:

Calories: 82, Fat: 7.6 g Carbs: 3.7, Fiber: 1.1 g, Protein: 1.2

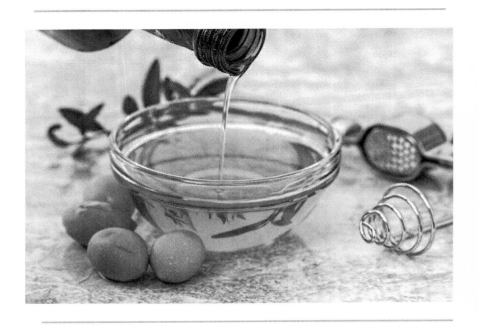

Homemade Salad Dressings

Warm Bacon Dressing

Serves 6 | PREP 10 min | COOK: 0 min | READY in: 10 min

INGREDIENTS

2 slices crumbled bacon

2 tbps. Bacon fat

2 tbsp. of Dijon mustard

4 tbsp. of red wine vinegar

2 small shallot chopped up very finely

2 tbps. Olive Oil

Salt and pepper to taste

DIRECTIONS

1. Drain bacon grease from grilled bacon (you could then use the bacon in your salad)
2. Whisk together the mustard and vinegar.
3. Gently fry the shallots until softened
4. Add the shallots to the mixture, and stir in the bacon fat. Add salt and pepper to taste.
5. Serve immediately, while hot.
6. This will store in the refrigerator for three days, and can be reheated before serving.

NUTRITION PER SERVING:

Calories: 45, Fat: 3.5 g Carbs: 0.5, Fiber: 0.2 g, Protein: 2.6

Mexi-Ranch Dressing

Serves **8** | Prep **10 min** | Cook: **0 min** | Ready in: **10 min**

INGREDIENTS

1 Cup Ranch Dressing (reduced fat)
1 tsp. cumin
1 tsp. chili powder
2 tbps. Hot sauce (or more to taste)

DIRECTIONS

Simply whisk the ingredients together and store in a glass jar in the fridge.

Nutrition Per Serving:

Calories: **58**, Fat: **5.1 g** Carbs: **2.4**, Fiber: **1 g**, Protein **0.3**

Balsamic Vinaigrette

Serves 10 | Prep 10 min | Cook: 0 min | Ready in: 10 min

INGREDIENTS

1/2 c. olive oil
1/2 c. Balsamic Vinegar
2 tbsp. grated parmesan
¼ tsp. Salt
½ tsp. Italian Seasoning
¼ tsp. Garlic Powder
¼ tsp. Black Pepper

DIRECTIONS

Simply Whisk the ingredients together. Store at room temperature and shake well before using.

Nutrition Per Serving:

Calories: **98,** Fat: **10.1 g** Carbs: **2.2,** Fiber: **0 g,** Protein **0.1**

Simple Healthy Dressing

Serves 2 | Prep 10 min | Cook: 0 min | Ready in: 10 min

INGREDIENTS

1tbsp. lemon
1/2 Tbsp. Olive oil
Salt and Pepper to Taste

DIRECTIONS

Simply Whisk the ingredients together. Store at room temperature and shake well before using.

Nutrition Per Serving:

Calories: 60, Fat: 7 g Carbs: 0, Fiber: 0 g, Protein0

Sweet & Tangy Italian

Serves 10 | Prep 10 min | Cook: 0 min | Ready in: 10 min

INGREDIENTS

3 Tablespoons Apple Cider vinegar
1 tsp Dijon mustard
1/4 cup olive oil
1/2 tsp onion powder
1-2 cloves finely minced garlic
1 tbsp. Italian Seasoning
½ tbsp. honey
½ tsp. Salt
¼ Tsp. Black pepper

DIRECTIONS

Whisk together ingredients and store in a sealed glass jar at room temperature. Shake very well before using (at least 30 seconds).

Nutrition Per Serving:

Calories: 53, Fat: 5.5g, Carbs: 1.3, Fiber: 0.1 g, Protein 0.1

Made in the
USA
Middletown, DE